The New Guide to
MASSAGE

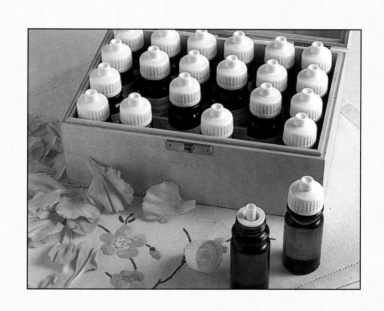

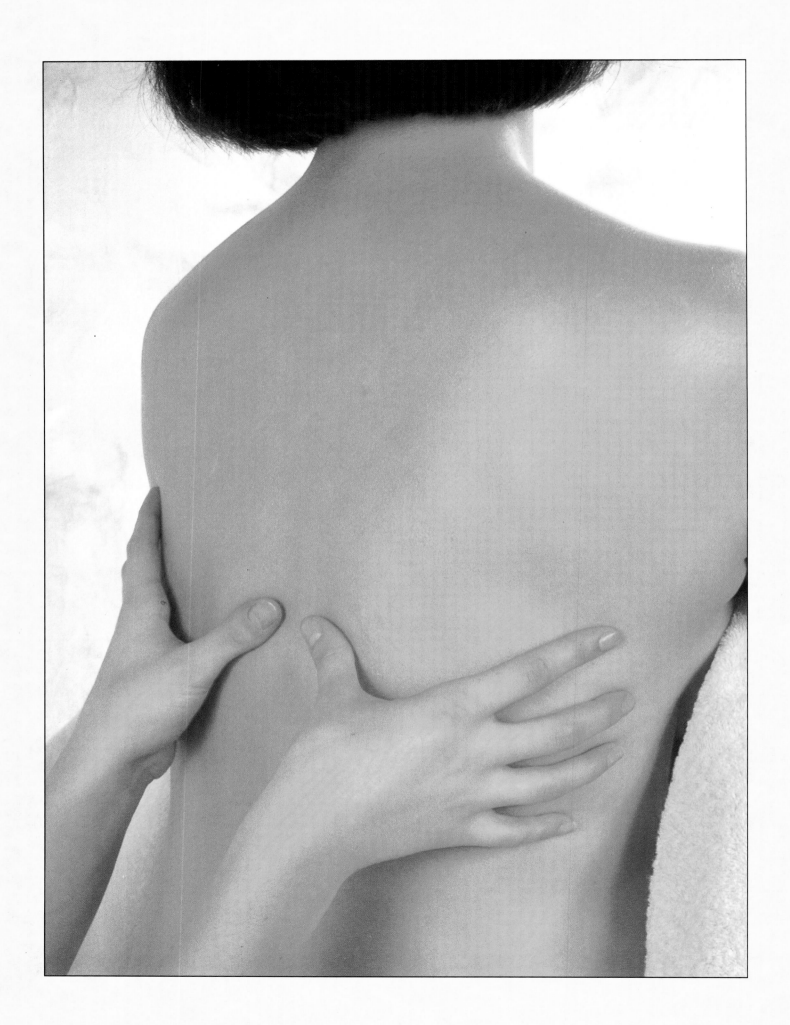

THE NEW GUIDE TO
MASSAGE

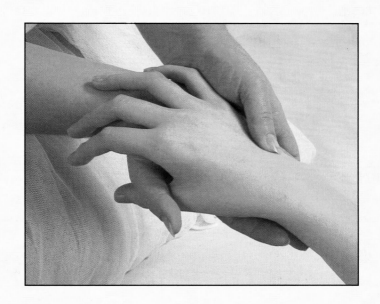

Photography by
SUE ATKINSON

LORENZ BOOKS
LONDON • NEW YORK • SYDNEY • BATH

First published in 1996 by Lorenz Books

Lorenz Books is an imprint of
Anness Pubishing Limited
1 Boundary Row
London SE1 8HP

This edition exclusively distributed
in Canada by Book Express
an imprint of
Raincoast Books Distribution Limited

ISBN 1 85967 194 2

Publisher: Joanna Lorenz
Project editor: Elaine Collins
Photography: Sue Atkinson
Photographic assistant: Kirsty Wilson
Designer: Kit Johnson
Jacket design: Adrian Morris
Artwork: Raymond Turvey, King & King
Typesetting by Dorchester Typesetting Group Ltd

Printed in Singapore by Star Standard Industries Pte. Ltd.

ACKNOWLEDGEMENTS

The authors and publishers would like to thank the following for their
valuable contributions to this book:

Kay Kiernan, Lisa Myhill, Karin Weisensel and Janice Welch, The
Bluestone Clinic and Henlow Grange for providing advice, expertise
and personnel.

Boutique Descampes, Culpeper, Decleor Ltd., Futon, Gore Booker,
Knickerbox, Kobashi, Pineapple Dance Studio and Purves and Purves for
providing equipment, clothes and products.

Juliet Algie, Andrea Ashley, Mary Atkinson, Alison Barry, Nichola Clare,
Paula Clark, Max Collins Wolff, Karen Flynn, Maya Jacobson, Maria
Johnson, Colette Keogh, Lisa Myhill, Sue Paterson-Jones, Anna Rand,
Michelle Thomas, Karin Weisensel, Janice Welch and Karen Wilding for
appearing in the photographs.

Previously published as *Step by Step Massage* and as part of a larger compendium
The Encyclopedia of Aromatherapy Massage and Yoga

PICTURE CREDITS

The Ancient Art and Architecture Collection: pp. 8 and 9.

CONTENTS

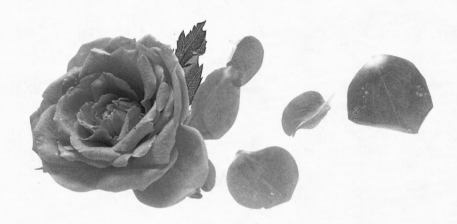

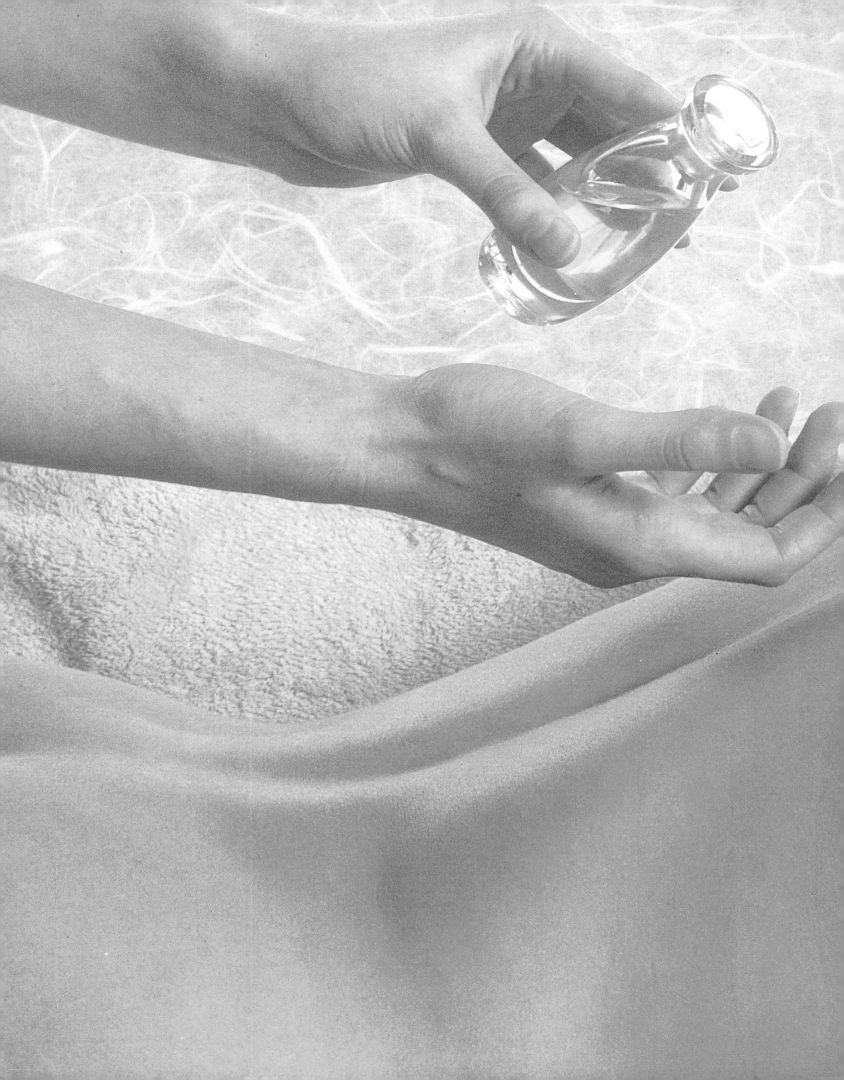

MASSAGE

Everyone enjoys massage. From babies to the elderly, from sportsmen and women to friends and lovers, all can benefit from this powerful form of communication. An effective aid to relaxation, massage helps to smoothe away stress, unknotting tense and aching muscles, relieving headaches and helping sleep problems. But massage is also invigorating: it improves the functioning of many of the body's systems, promotes healing and tones muscles, leaving you with a feeling of renewed energy. By mastering a few simple techniques and sequences, you will learn the language of touch – a valuable gift for yourself and others.

THE HUMAN TOUCH

The sense of touch is a powerful and highly sensitive form of communication. It is a natural reaction to reach out and touch, whether to feel the shape or texture of something, or to respond to another person, perhaps by comforting them. A mother cuddles her baby, family pets are stroked, sexual partners caress, and if we accidentally knock a limb we instinctively "rub it better".

To touch someone can mean various things in different cultures. There are many social restraints which inhibit touching in public. For us, a formal handshake, nod of the head, and even a peck on each cheek are all recognized forms of greeting, and yet you can carry them out without showing any real emotion. Indeed, our rather formal approach to physical contact is contrary to our most basic instincts and needs. Fortunately, we are now rediscovering the healing power of massage and other touch therapies which have been understood in other cultures for thousands of years.

THE DEVELOPMENT OF MASSAGE

History shows that although the early Egyptians made references to the benefits of massage, the Chinese were among the first to recognize its healing value at around 3000 BC. Roman and Greek philosophers and physicians prescribed it both for its restorative powers after battle and for general preservation of the body and mind. Although the Romans believed in its curative powers, the art of massage also became part of a daily ritual for relaxation. After bathing, oils would be used to anoint the body from head to toe, followed by a luxurious massage.

Herbalists throughout history have used massage to heal body and soul, both by applying balms and by laying their own hands on the afflicted to expel evil spirits and clear the mind. It wasn't until the eighteenth and nineteenth centuries, though, that massage became popular throughout Europe, thanks to the work of Per Henrik Ling (1776–1839). Ling was a Swede who travelled to China and returned with a detailed insight into their massage techniques. From these he developed his own system of massage based on a variety of movements, involving pressure, friction, vibration and rotation.

This wealth of practical knowledge soon spread, and medical and non-medical professions worldwide began exploring the benefits of massage. This eventually established the basis of massage today, which in many ways remains much the same now as those early Swedish techniques.

Along with basic massage we are now experiencing a

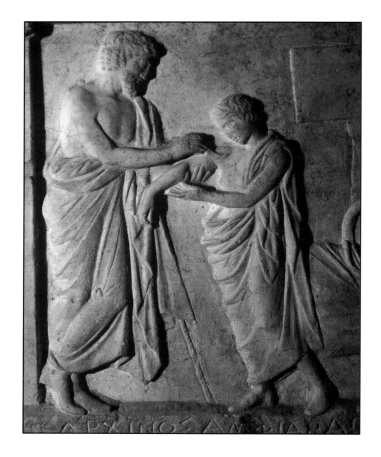

revival of interest in many of the ancient arts which place such great importance on touch. These include aromatherapy, reflexology and shiatsu – all distinctive natural therapies which have a specific role to play in "alternative" health-care.

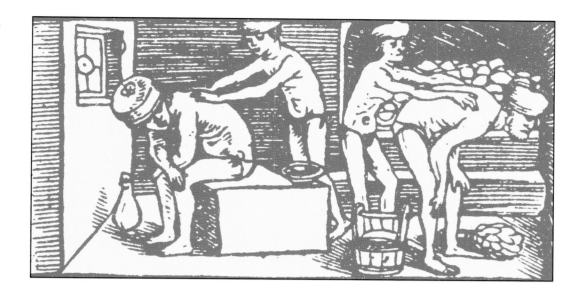

Below left: This Greek stone relief from the fourth century BC shows the physician Aesculapius treating a patient by "rubbing", as recommended by Hippocrates.

Right: As Europe emerged from the Middle Ages, massage once again became part of the bathing ritual, as shown in this sixteenth-century German woodcut of a public bath house.

EFFECTS OF MASSAGE

Massage can stimulate and relax the body and the mind. The skin, blood and lymphatic systems are stimulated, which boosts circulation, aids cellular renewal and removes toxic wastes. As tense muscles relax, stiff joints loosen and nerves are soothed, an all-over feeling of relaxation and well-being comes about.

The Nervous System
The nervous system is a highly complex network which relays messages from the brain to the rest of the body. The part of the nervous system which regulates many physiological functions leaves the brain at the base of the skull and runs down the spinal cord, protected by the spine's bony vertebrae. Millions of nerve endings run throughout the body, controlling much of the way it functions. Depending on the depth of the massage movements used, the nerve endings can be stimulated or soothed.

The Skin
With massage comes an increase in blood circulation. This helps the exfoliation of superficial dead skin cells, tones the skin and encourages its renewal process. Massage helps maintain the collagen fibres, which give skin its elasticity and strength, and keep wrinkles at bay. The activity of the sweat and sebaceous glands, which lubricate and moisturize the skin, is regulated.

Muscles
With the increase in blood flow, the blood's vital nutrients circulate more efficiently. Massage is popular with sportsmen and women because it can improve muscle tone, restore mobility, and ensure the elimination of waste products after exercise. With regular massage, strains and sprains heal more rapidly, while calf cramps and stiff muscles can become a thing of the past. Massage before an exercise session will help loosen and warm up the muscles, or afterwards it will ease sore, aching limbs.

Circulation and Lymphatic Systems
By dilating the blood vessels, massage increases the blood circulation. A good circulatory system means that an efficient supply of the blood's constituents, including oxygen and nutrients, reaches the billions of individual cells. This is vital for the healthy functioning of the whole body, from the muscles to internal organs such as the kidneys and liver.

At the same time the increase in blood circulation helps accelerate the lymphatic system, which absorbs and eliminates waste substances. Unlike the blood circulation, which has the heart to pump it round, the lymphatic system has no pump of its own and is dependent on muscular action for its efficiency. Massage is an important means of speeding up the flow of the lymph, encouraging a more effective filtering and elimination of waste throughout the body. An efficient lymphatic system provides the body with a strong immune system to fight against infections and disease.

Digestion
Massage mobilizes the digestive system so that the processes of assimilation and elimination are improved, helping problems like constipation and flatulence. The digestive system is quick to respond to stress, and the reduction in anxiety and tension which comes with regular massage has a regulating effect on the digestion.

THE BASIC TECHNIQUES

When many people think of massage they picture the vigorous pummelling and slapping often associated with puritanical health spas. In truth, firm massage can be highly beneficial without causing discomfort. Alternate firm and gentle flowing strokes to create a combination that will alleviate tension and muscular aches and pains whilst energizing and invigorating the body.

In Swedish massage there are four basic types of movement. Familiarize yourself with these different techniques before beginning the step-by-step, whole-body massage.

EFFLEURAGE

Effleurage describes long, soothing, stroking movements using the flat of the hand (or fingers if working on small areas). These are often used to apply oil evenly to the body. You can use one hand on its own or with the other providing support on top of it, both hands simultaneously, or one hand alternating with the other.

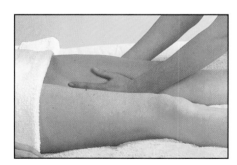

Relax the hands and mould them to the contours of the body. Apply slightly more pressure when you take the stroke in the direction of the heart to improve circulation and lymph flow. If you are working away from the heart, keep the pressure firmer on the return stroke. The movements should be fairly slow and continuous. Keep the hands in contact with your partner between strokes.

Effleurage is used to start off a massage, soothing the nerve endings and helping your partner get used to your touch. It is used again at the end of a massage for a relaxing finish. In between, *effleurage* movements provide an important link between other more stimulating strokes and are used to make first contact with a new area of the body. If you feel hesitant about what to do next, you can always insert some *effleurage*, so the continuity is not lost.

You repeat *effleurage* strokes several times. Each time try to start the first complete stroke with fairly light pressure, then apply slightly more pressure with the next complete stroke. Where there are larger muscle areas, such as the thighs and back, you can apply the most pressure for a more stimulating effect.

PETRISSAGE

Petrissage describes a number of movements which involve various ways of kneading, rolling and picking up the skin and muscles. These firm and strengthen the structures by stimulating the deep layers of tissue, and increasing the supply of blood to the area. They also improve the flow of lymph.

Generally a single group of muscles, or an individual muscle, is worked on at one time. The basic kneading action is very similar to kneading dough.

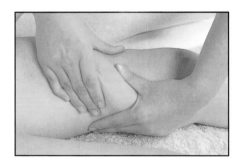

For *petrissage*, start with your fingers pointing away from you, press down with the palm, grasp the flesh between fingers and thumb and push it toward the other hand. As you release the first hand your second hand grasps the flesh and pushes it back toward the first hand. It is a continuous action, alternating the hands to squeeze and release.

With light kneading you are tackling the top muscle layers, whilst firmer kneading works on the deeper muscles, easing taut muscles and breaking down congested tissues to help the elimination of waste products.

10

FRICTION

Friction, or "connective tissue massage", is a penetrating circular movement which applies deep direct pressure to one particular site of muscular tension, using the thumb, fingertips or knuckles. It is a valuable technique for concentrating on specific areas of tightness and muscle spasm in the back.

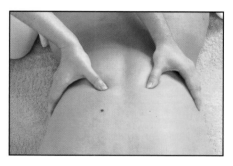

As you make the circular rotations you should actually feel the underlying tissues moving; you are not simply sliding over the skin's surface.

A variation on circular friction pressures is static pressure, where you lean gradually into the muscle, slowly deepening the pressure without the rotation action. Press for a few seconds, then gradually release.

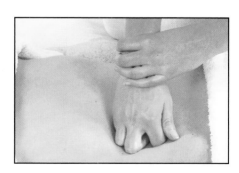

Another friction movement is knuckling: use the knuckles in a loosely clenched fist to produce rippling, circular motions. This is used to release tension up the sides of the spine and in other areas. Remember not to work right on top of the spine bone.

TAPOTEMENT

Tapotement, or percussion movements, are fast and stimulating. They include cupping, hacking, pounding (also called pummelling), which all sound like painful practices but when carried out properly should certainly not cause bruising or pain. (Don't use *tapotement* on particularly bony areas or on broken or varicose veins.) For all the movements, remember to keep the hands and wrists relaxed. All the percussion techniques are fast, precision actions, bringing one hand quickly after the other into contact with your partner. It is particularly important at the beginning to ask your partner whether you are applying the right degree of pressure.

These sequences stimulate the blood circulation, tone and help strengthen sagging skin and muscles. In particular *tapotement* can tighten up soft tissue areas, such as thighs and buttocks, which are prone to cellulite.

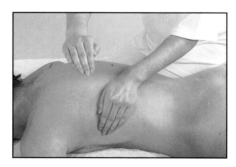

For cupping, gently curve the hands to make a loose cupped shape, bending at the knuckles while keeping the fingers straight and firm. Do not bend the fingers too far over. Using the cupped palm, make a bouncy, brisk, cupping action against a fleshy area, alternating the hands quickly. The fast, cupping action creates a suction against the skin. Try this movement on the back, buttocks and thighs.

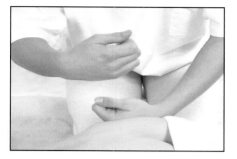

For pounding (or pummelling), loosely clench your fists, but keep the wrists relaxed. You can use the wrists in two ways: either striking your partner with the outer edges of the loose fist or with the front of the knuckles. Either way, the speed and rhythm of the movement is similar: brisk and firm, alternating the hands, without thumping your partner too enthusiastically. Once again, keep to the fleshier parts of the body, particularly cellulite zones such as hips, buttocks and thighs.

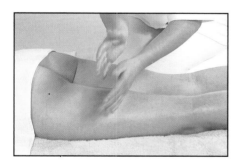

In hacking, the outer edge of the hand is used to stimulate the area by striking it quickly with alternate hands. You need to practise a brisk, bouncing movement, working rhythmically and rapidly over a fleshy area of the body. You need to have very relaxed wrists and fingers, and use the sides of the palm rather than the fingers. Used over the buttocks and thighs, hacking tones up muscles and disperses fluid.

Intersperse these brisk movements with the gentler, *effleurage* strokes, then go back to the pounding or pummelling for as long as you both feel comfortable.

WHOLE-BODY MASSAGE

Our whole-body massage is a comprehensive, top-to-toe sequence based on Swedish massage techniques, specially adapted for home practice. As a beginner you may find the full sequence too tiring at first. Until your hands and wrists build up their strength and you get used to positioning your own body comfortably to perform the massage, it is best to work on just a few parts of the body, such as the back of the legs, back and shoulders, or to perform fewer movements on each part of the body. Your partner will find it more relaxing if you perform one or two types of movement thoroughly rather than keep changing the strokes after a few seconds to cover all the steps. Always include *effleurage* strokes to begin and end a sequence, and never leave the body unbalanced – if you work on one leg or arm, you should repeat the same movements on the other side of the body.

COMFORT AND CLOTHING

If you are going to massage on the floor, put down a thick layer of blankets or towels, or a futon, to provide your partner with a firm, comfortable cushion. There is nothing more likely to reverse the relaxation process than a hard surface, a cold room and noise. Choose a quiet time, when you won't be disturbed. Your partner may need the room quite a lot warmer than you might expect. Being massaged on the floor might be extremely comfortable for your partner, but it can put a strain on the masseur's back and knees so, if you prefer, set up the same cushioning surface on a large table. It is not a good idea to massage on a bed – the give of a soft mattress can counteract much of your effort.

Have ready several towels, so that you can cover areas of the body which are not being worked on. Often a sense of modesty is crucial to relaxation, and the towels will also keep your partner warm. Move the towels around to cover most of the body, and especially an area you have just

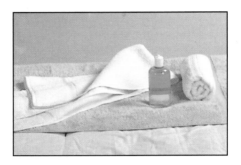

finished working on. You will need a cushion or towel to support the head, and it can be helpful to put a roll of towel under the knees when your partner is lying on their back. This relaxes the lower back. When your partner turns over on to the front, a towel under the chest can improve comfort.

Massage in loose-fitting clothes, with soft-soled, flat shoes, or work in bare feet. Take off rings and jewellery, so there is nothing to distract your partner, and make sure your nails are short! The more relaxed you are, as the masseur, the better. If you feel keyed up, try some deep, regular breathing exercises before you start. Take a few stretches, shake your hands to loosen any tension, and you're ready to start.

OILS

There are several oils which are appropriate for body massage. Stick to vegetable oils, rather than mineral oils such as baby oil. Grapeseed, sunflower or almond oil are good, basic vegetable oils, which are light and therefore not too sticky. Jojoba is a good oil for the face, especially if your partner has oily skin. Avoid oils with strong smells, such as olive oil. Also try experimenting by adding a little avocado, apricot or peach kernel oil if you wish, or buy ready-mixed massage oil.

Measure 3–4 tablespoons (45–60 ml) oil into a saucer or small container before starting your massage. You will quickly get used to how much oil to apply. The amount varies with the dryness of the skin, and how readily it absorbs the oil, but in general you need enough to facilitate the strokes without applying so much that your hands simply slide over the skin. If you need to apply more oil during a sequence, simply smooth a little oil into the palms of your hands and do some extra *effleurage* strokes.

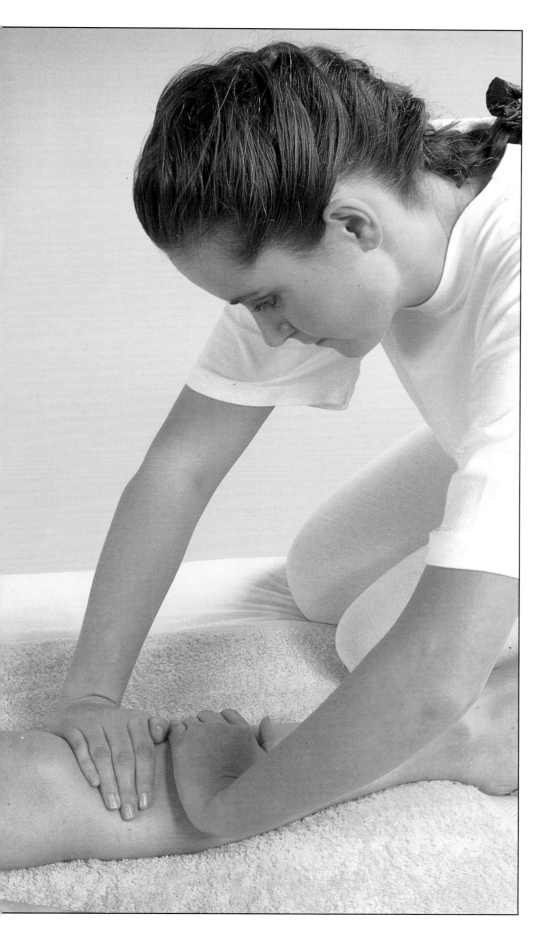

Exchanging a regular basic massage is a luxury for both giver and receiver. However, specific problems should be tackled by a trained practitioner. Never massage right on top of the spine. Working down each side of the bony spinal column is fine, and produces many benefits, but you should avoid working directly on top of the spine.

There are occasions when it is not appropriate to massage. Avoid if there are any of the following conditions:

- heart condition
- high blood pressure
- bacterial or viral infection
- nausea or abdominal pain
- severe back pain which may be caused by the spine, especially if there are shooting pains in other limbs
- temperature or fever
- open wound or skin infection
- cancer
- post-operative recovery

If you are in any doubt, it is always best to check with your doctor first.

THE FULL MASSAGE SEQUENCE

Front of Body:
1 Legs 2 Feet and ankles
3 Arms and hands 4 Chest, shoulders and neck 5 Face
6 Abdomen and waist
Back of Body:
7 Legs and buttocks
8 Back and shoulders

FRONT OF BODY

*The full massage begins with the front of the body, so your partner should
lie face up with cushions or rolled towels wherever needed for support.*

LEGS

*Since legs carry the full body weight, the bones and
muscles in the legs are the largest and strongest we
have. A good leg massage can not only help to relieve
strain and tension in the legs, but can benefit the well-
being of the whole body. It's not unknown for backache
to be traced to problems in the legs, and for a good leg
massage to help alleviate the pain.*

*Leg massage stimulates both the blood circulation
and the lymphatic system, and done regularly it helps to
prevent varicose veins. Any congestion in the lower legs
will be lessened with* effleurage *movements taken up
toward the lymph nodes at the back of the knee and in
the groin. If legs feel puffy or swollen to the touch,
make sure you use the gentlest of pressure. Firm
massage on the larger muscles, such as those round the
thighs, can dispel tiredness and stimulate a sluggish
lymphatic system. Work more lightly over bony areas
such as the shins and knees.*

═══ VARICOSE VEINS ═══

You need to take certain precautions
if your partner has varicose veins.
Never knead or put any pressure on
varicose veins, and only massage the
part of the leg which is higher than
the area with veins (that is, only
massage closer to the heart); never on
or below the vein.

EFFLEURAGE

1 *Below: Kneel beside your
partner's left ankle. With a
little oil in the palm of your hands,
start with your hands crossed over
the ankle, in readiness to begin
several long effleurage strokes. You
will need more oil if the legs are
particularly hairy or dry, but don't
add too much in the first instance.*

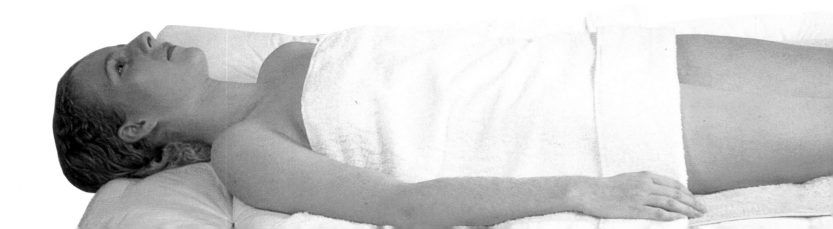

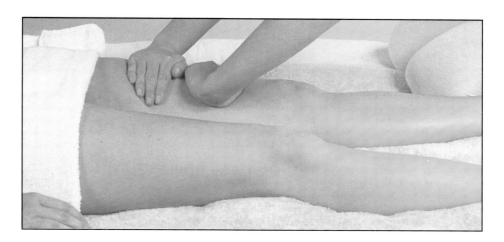

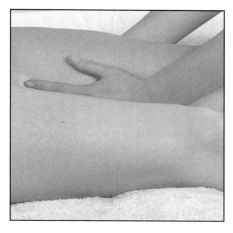

2 *Keeping your hands crossed over the leg, slide the palms up the front of the leg, over the knee and up to the thigh, in one continuous, sweeping movement to oil the front of the leg evenly.*

3 *Turn the hands outward round the hip, separate them and bring the hands back down each side of the thigh.*

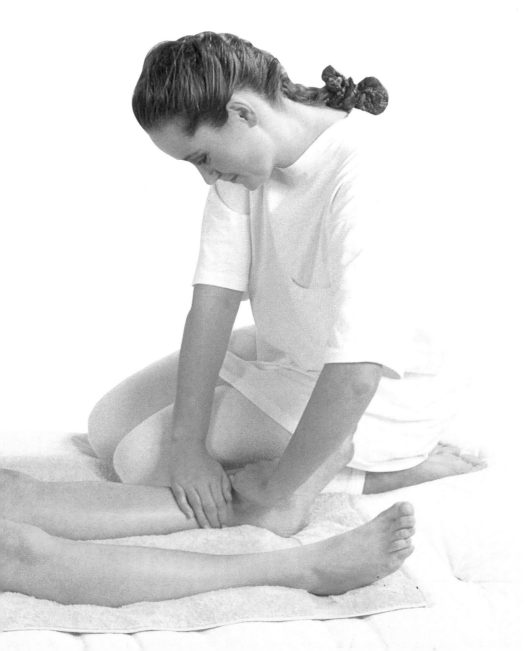

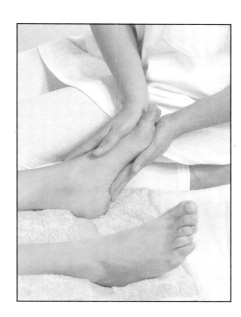

4 *Continue to sweep the hands back to the ankle, and then over the foot to the toes. Then place your hands crossed over the ankle again, ready to repeat the entire movement.*

Use some more oil if necessary, and this time use slightly firmer pressure on the upward stroke, then lighter again for the return. The stroke is smooth and continuous throughout.

Repeat the sequence over the whole leg once again.

THIGHS

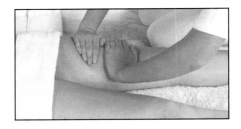

1 Bring both hands up to just above the knee and move them up together, pressing the muscles firmly toward the upper thigh. You should be applying enough pressure to see movement in the muscles.

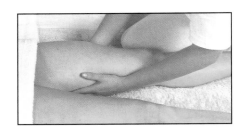

2 At the top of the thigh separate the hands and using lighter pressure come down either side of the leg to the knee.

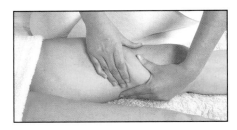

3 Begin kneading the inner thigh with both hands. Squeeze, then release the muscles, picking up and rolling them as you do so. Continue the kneading action over the top and outside thigh.

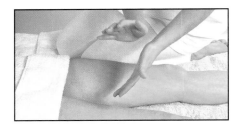

4 Now use a hacking movement all over the thigh. Briskly strike the area with the outside edge of one hand after another, using short, sharp movements. Keep a fast repetition going.

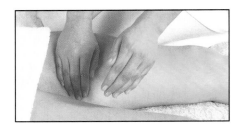

5 Continue with cupping all over the thigh, working quickly. Expect quite a loud cupping sound, but check with your partner that the strokes are not too powerful.

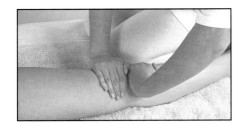

6 Begin at the knee and do some effleurage strokes up to the top of the thigh, sweeping the hands outward and back down to the knee, to soothe the area after the series of stimulating movements.

KNEES

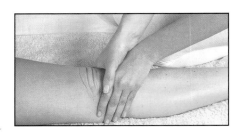

1 Place both hands just below the knee. Lightly massage round the kneecap, using your fingertips to work gently into the muscles. Repeat three times.

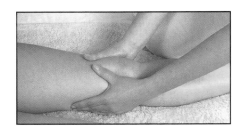

2 Starting with your thumbs above the kneecap, with your hands under the knee for support, slowly draw them lightly round the outside of the kneecap and release. Repeat this movement three times.

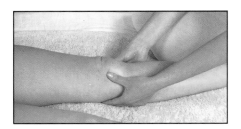

3 Support the back of the knee with your hands and use your thumbs to circle gently round the kneecap, working downward. Return to the top of the knee and repeat three times.

4 *Right: Raise the height of your hands above the knee. Work round the kneecap with one hand, loosening the muscles with your thumb and fingers. Use gentle, circular rotations to cover the area thoroughly.*

You may find it easier to support your wrist with the other hand.

Do some more effleurage *strokes, sweeping them up from the ankle to just below the kneecap and back down to the ankle. Repeat this several times.*

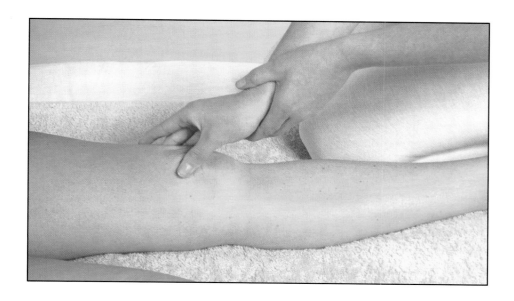

CALVES

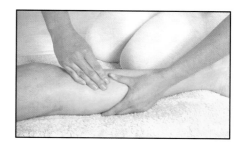

1 *Knead the calf muscles. Squeeze and release them, working from the ankle up to the knee.*

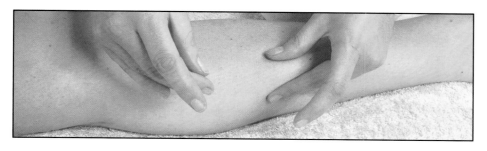

2 *Lightly and quickly pinch the fleshy part of the calf with the fingers and thumbs, one hand after the other. Check with your* partner that you are not pinching too hard, although this needs to be felt to be effective.

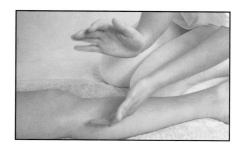

3 *Using the outside edge of both hands, alternately and rhythmically strike the calf muscles, working up and down the entire length, but keeping away from the bony shin area itself. Keep the hacking action short and brisk.*

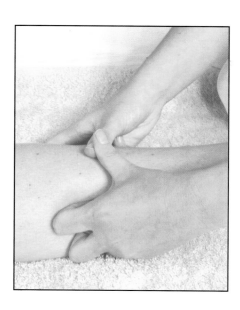

4 *Left: Starting at the ankle and crossing your thumbs on top of the shin for support, with loose knuckles make semi-circular kneading movements, working up and down the calf.*

Finish the leg with some effleurage *movements from ankle to thigh.*

FEET AND ANKLES

A foot massage is particularly relaxing after the legs have been worked on. It can alleviate anxiety and stress, stimulate the circulation and nervous system, help insomniacs to sleep, and energize anyone feeling tired and lethargic. There are thousands of nerve endings in the foot, particularly on the sole. Try to include the ankles too, to improve their flexibility.

Change the pressure of the strokes to suit your partner, remembering that deeper pressure tends to revitalize whereas gentle strokes increase relaxation throughout the entire person. When working on the feet it is best to use only a very little oil, otherwise your hands will slide around and tickle. If your partner's feet are hot and sticky, use a little talcum powder instead.

Before starting, you may wish to raise your partner's knee slightly with a rolled towel under them, to relax the muscles around the knee and in the lower back.

FEET AND ANKLES

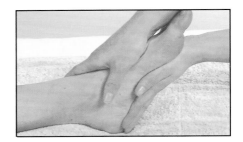

1 *Kneel at your partner's feet. Starting with the hands at the ankle, gently slide your hands toward the tips of the toes and then release them. Repeat several times. If you are using oil, apply it with this stroke.*

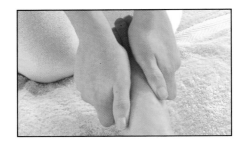

2 *With the heels of your hand, give a good stretch to the top of the foot. Draw the heel toward the sides of the foot to give the stretch. Repeat a few times, working slightly further down the foot too.*

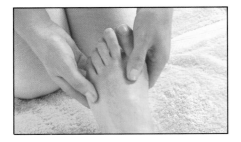

3 *Supporting the foot in both hands, find the furrow between each tendon and, using small, circular movements, work both thumbs up the tendons toward the ankle. Repeat three times on each tendon.*

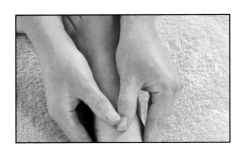

4 *Resting the thumbs across the top of the ankle, work the fingers right round the ankle bone using light, circular movements.*

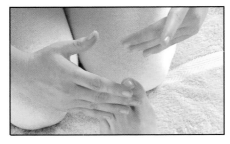

5 *Lightly tap the toes with your fingers to build up some gentle friction.*

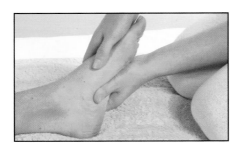

6 *Now knead the foot firmly, working particularly well into the arch. You will need to use different parts of the hand, such as the heel, knuckle and thumbs.*

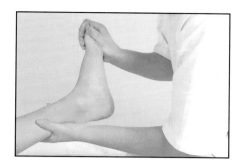

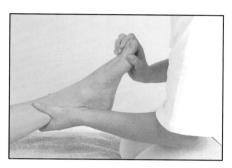

7, 8 *Supporting the lower leg with your left hand, gently rotate the ankle three times in each direction, without forcing.*

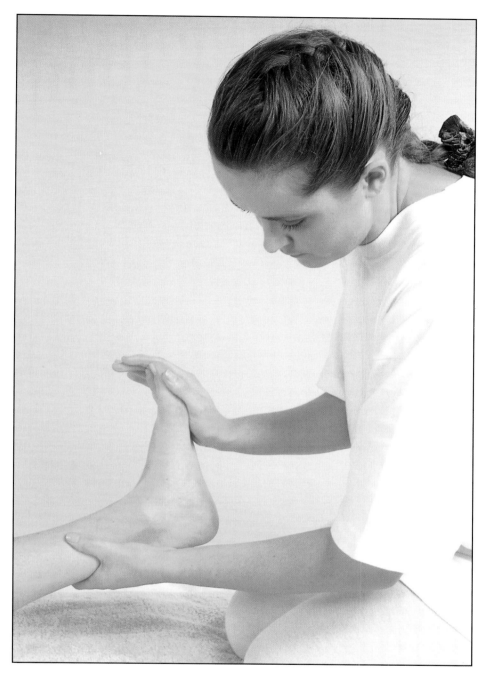

9 *Right: Give the foot a gentle stretch backward and forward, to relax and flex the tendons. Supporting the back of the lower leg, use your other hand at the toes to push the foot gently away from you. To reverse the stretch take the hand over the top of the foot, and press the foot down, still supporting the lower leg with the other hand.*

10 *Finish the foot and ankle sequence with some long sweeping, effleurage strokes from the top of the foot up the lower leg and back down to the foot, to help reintegrate the foot and the leg. Repeat several times, varying the pressure.*

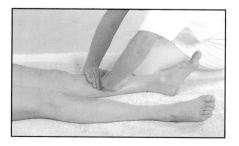

Move round your partner to kneel on the other side.
Repeat the entire sequence on the front of the other leg and the other foot.

ARMS AND HANDS

Arms and hands can hide the most powerful emotions. Tight, clenched arms and hands often reflect insecurity, self-protection and unresolved anger. Whether the posture is intentional or sub-conscious, tension in the arms can cause headaches, neck pain, and aching shoulders. Don't be put off if your partner's arms are slim and bony, there are still important muscle areas there.

A hand massage feels surprisingly good, almost on a par with having the feet massaged. A lot of tension creeps into the hands: a massage is a reminder of how it feels to relax them. Massaging the arms and hands can liberate and relax not only the muscles but also the pent-up emotions, as your partner starts to feel the wonderful sensation of letting go.

ARMS

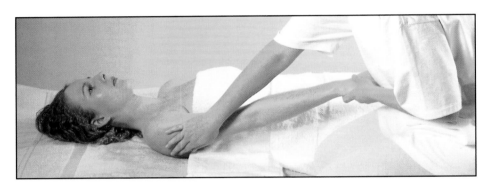 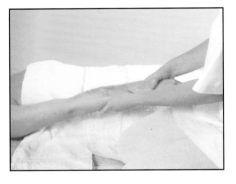

1 *Kneel halfway along your partner's right side. Holding the wrist with your left hand, lightly oil the arm using* effleurage *strokes, starting from the wrist and sweeping your hand up round the shoulder and down again. Repeat three times.*

2 *Changing hands, so that your partner's wrist is supported in your right hand, use the left hand to stroke gently from the wrist to the shoulder, and back down again. Repeat several times.*

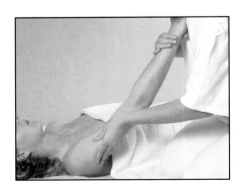 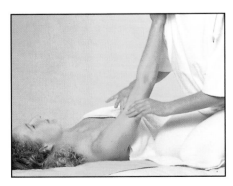 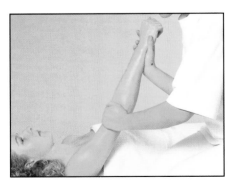

3 *Lift the arm and rest the hand on your right shoulder ready to start kneading. Support your partner's wrist with your left hand and use your right to knead lightly the muscles of the upper arm, working from elbow to shoulder.*

4 *Keeping your partner's hand supported by your shoulder, use the fingers of both hands to continue the kneading.*

5 *Still holding the arm across the front of your chest with your right hand, do some* effleurage *strokes from the elbow up to the shoulder and back down again. Repeat three times.*

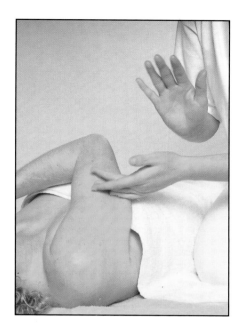

6 Bend your partner's arm and rest the right hand on the left shoulder. Using the outside edge of your hands, do some short, brisk hacking on the outer and under sides of the arm.

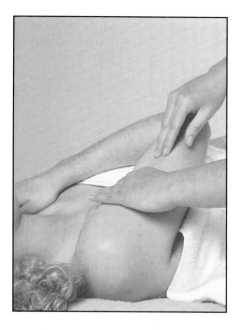

7 With your partner's arm still bent, firmly knead the muscles of the upper arm with your right hand, using the left hand to keep your partner's arm stable.

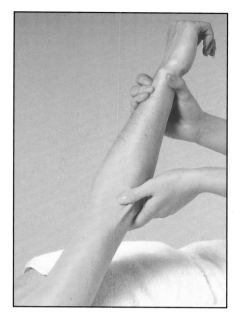

8 Holding the wrist for support with your right hand, work round the outside of the elbow with your fingers and thumb, using smooth circular movements and covering the area thoroughly. As the elbows can get particularly dry you may need some more oil.

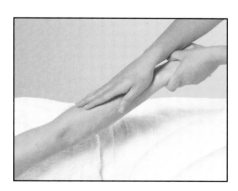

9 To encourage further relaxation, hold the wrist with the left hand and do some effleurage strokes up and down the top of the forearm. Keep the pressure fairly firm.

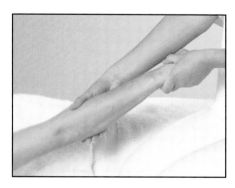

10 Repeat these effleurage strokes on the inside of the forearm.

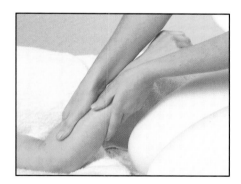

11 Rest your partner's elbow back on the towel. Supporting the weight of the lower arm in your left hand, use your right hand to knead the inside of the forearm, starting from the wrist. When you reach the elbow glide gently back to the wrist to begin again. Repeat three times.

Finish the arm with a few effleurage strokes and then massage the hand and wrist (see the following pages) before moving on to the other arm.

HANDS AND WRISTS

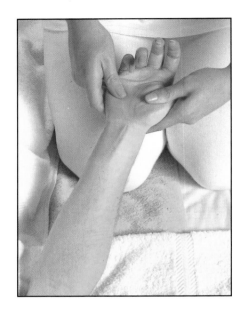

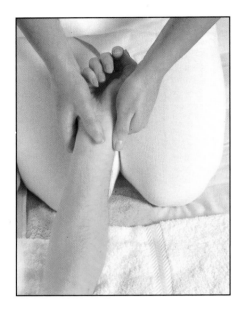

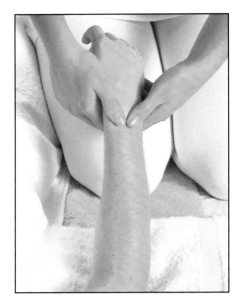

1 *Support your partner's hand in both hands and gently use the thumbs to knead the palm. This should be a continuous, circular action, with the thumbs alternately applying the pressure.*

2 *Rest your hands under your partner's wrist and use the thumbs to stroke outward round the wrist. Then work with the thumbs up the inner forearm toward the elbow, using circular movements.*

3 *Turn the hand over, supporting the wrist. Massage gently over the back of the wrist with your thumbs.*

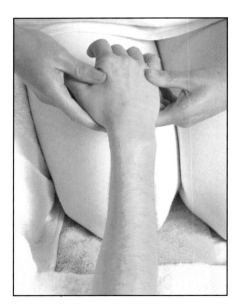

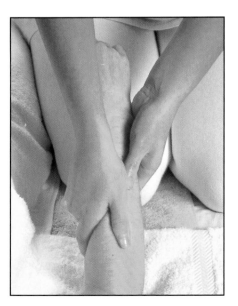

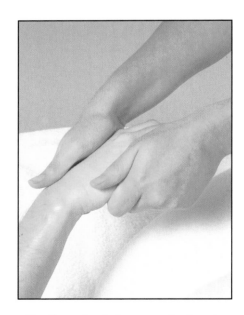

4 *Stroke up in between the tendons on the back of the hand with your thumbs, from knuckles to wrist, using light small circles. Repeat twice between each tendon.*

5 *Sweep the hands alternately up from the wrist toward the elbow, applying a fairly firm pressure with the inside edge of the hands. Repeat several times.*

6 *Come back down to the hand and stretch the back of the hand, drawing your hands out toward the sides.*

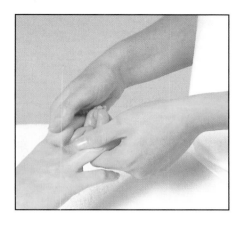

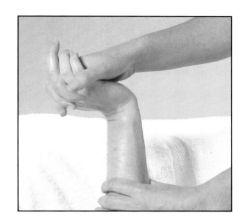

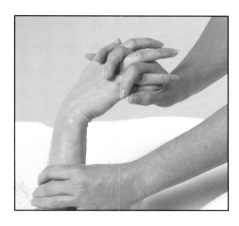

7 *With one hand make circular pressure movements round each of the three joints on each finger, starting at the tip. When you have worked round all three joints, gently rotate the finger twice. Then gently stretch each finger to release the joints.*

8 *Raising your partner's lower arm and supporting it with your left hand, clasp your partner's hand with your right hand, and gently rotate it in a half circle, three times in each direction.*

9 *Still supporting the lower arm, thread your fingers between your partner's and gently bend the wrist backward and forward three times, making sure that the wrist joint is not forced.*

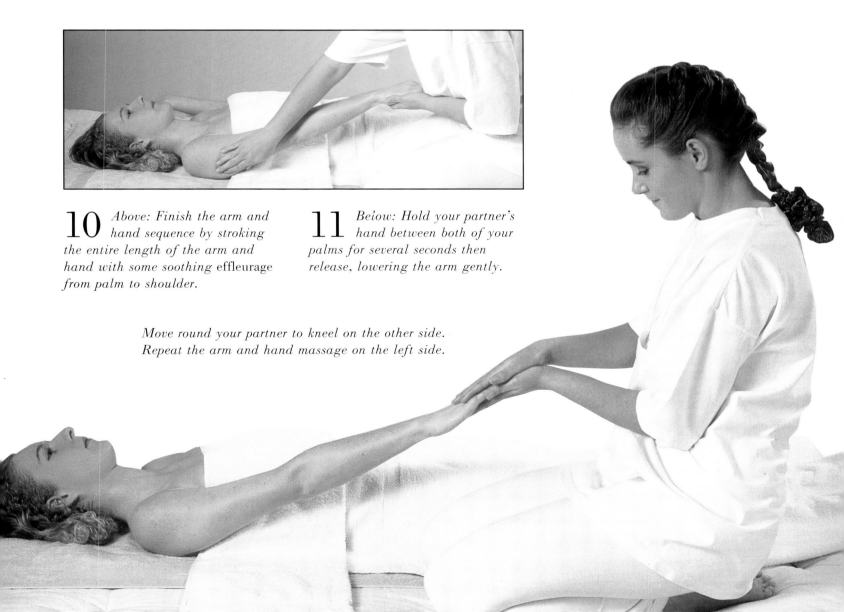

10 *Above: Finish the arm and hand sequence by stroking the entire length of the arm and hand with some soothing* effleurage *from palm to shoulder.*

11 *Below: Hold your partner's hand between both of your palms for several seconds then release, lowering the arm gently.*

Move round your partner to kneel on the other side. Repeat the arm and hand massage on the left side.

CHEST, SHOULDERS AND NECK

Ideally a chest massage should follow an arm massage and precede a facial massage. It's not only the hours spent sitting hunched over a desk that tighten and contract the chest muscles – clutching a car steering wheel, carrying heavy shopping, and poor posture all *have a cumulative effect. Tension in the chest can also exacerbate inflexibility and stiffness in the neck and the shoulders. We tend to raise the shoulders toward our ears, until they become set rigid with tension. This sequence includes work to help these problems.*

First check if your partner would be more comfortable with a small cushion or a folded towel under the head. They may or may not, but it is important that the neck should be comfortable. Kneel behind your partner's head to start the sequence.

CHEST

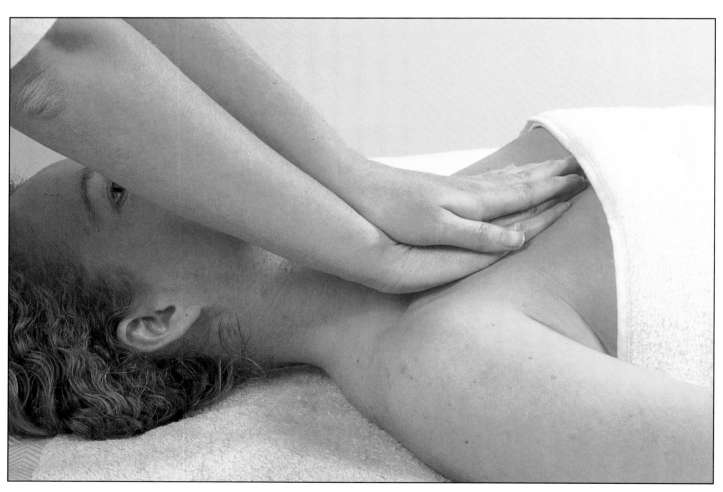

1 *Lightly oil the palm of your right hand, and with the flat of the hands placed on the chest. fingers pointing toward your* *partner's feet, place the left hand on top of the right. You will be doing reinforced* effleurage *on the right side of the chest first.*

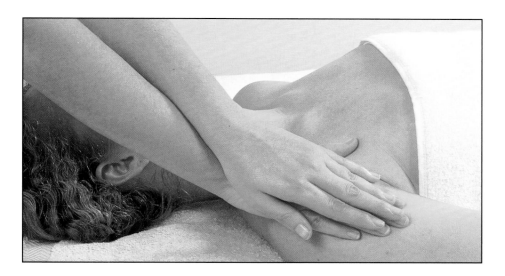

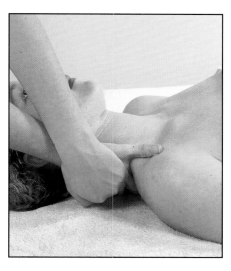

2 *Sweep your hands over the chest, toward and round the right shoulder, keeping the left hand over the right. The movement should be a continuous* effleurage *stroke. You should apply enough pressure to press the chest and shoulder toward the floor, so that they release as you lift off after the stroke. Repeat three times.*

3 *Continue the* effleurage *stroke, sweeping both hands round and up the right side of the neck.*

Repeat the sequence twice more, starting from the centre of the chest.

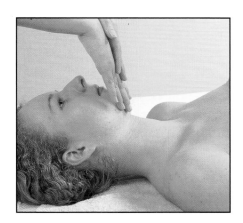

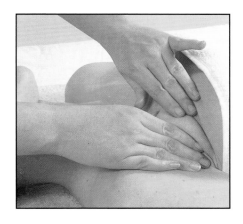

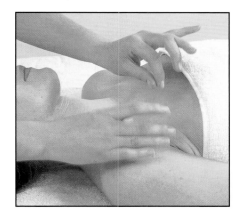

4 *Repeat the sequence once again, but this time finish by bringing both hands up to the jawline with the fingers resting lightly under the centre of the jaw.*

5 *With both hands, knead the fleshy area in front of the armpit. Pick up and release the muscles, squeezing them from one hand to the other.*

6 *On the same fleshy area, lightly pinch the surface muscles between the thumb and first finger. Alternate the hands swiftly in a rhythmical action, checking with your partner that there is no discomfort.*

Repeat the effleurage *strokes from the centre of the chest and over the right side of the neck in one continuous movement, to soothe the area you have worked on.*

Then repeat the entire sequence on the left side of the chest and neck, lightly oiling the palm of your left hand before you begin.

SHOULDERS AND NECK

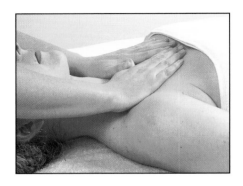

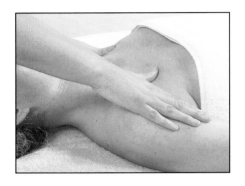

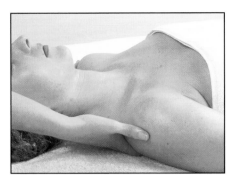

1 Place both hands fairly firmly, side by side, over the front of the chest.

2 Sweep them out toward each shoulder with firm effleurage strokes, taking them over the shoulders, round under the upper back and up the back of the neck.

3 When you take the movement round the back and the neck gently lift the weight of your partner to give the muscles a gentle stretch.

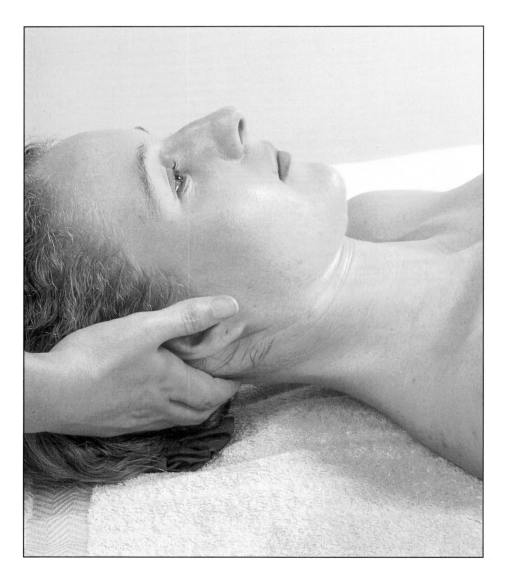

4 Left: With the fingertips, work with circular pressures up the back of the neck to the base of the skull. These should be small, firm rotations, which you can feel easing taut muscles. You should spend some time on this area, which is often extremely tense.

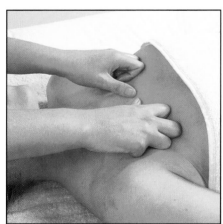

5 With loose fists, use the knuckle area to ripple your fingers in semi-circular frictions all over the upper chest. Keep the half circles fairly small and apply quite firm pressure on the fleshier area, but avoid working directly on the collarbone.

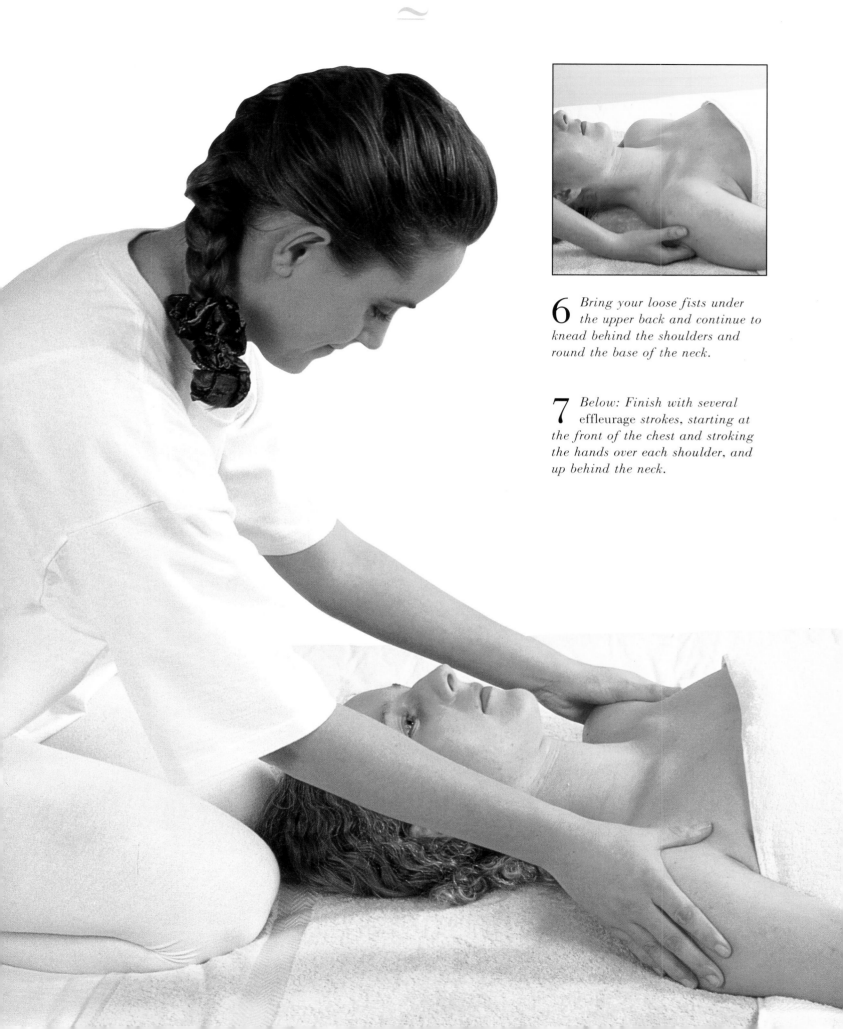

6 *Bring your loose fists under the upper back and continue to knead behind the shoulders and round the base of the neck.*

7 *Below: Finish with several effleurage strokes, starting at the front of the chest and stroking the hands over each shoulder, and up behind the neck.*

FACE

The face constantly mirrors our health and emotions. Stress and tension are reflected in a furrowed brow, and lines around the eyes, mouth and jawline. A face massage can soothe away headaches, anxiety and exhaustion and replace them with a feeling of serenity. It improves the circulation, giving the skin a healthy glow.

If your partner wears contact lenses make sure they are removed before you start a face massage. Use a little light facial oil, and don't let the oil get too near or in the eyes. Keep the hands relaxed. You may be surprised to find that the face is less fragile than it looks and you can apply quite deep pressure without discomfort.

Your partner will probably still prefer to have a small cushion or towel under the head. Use a towelling hairband to keep the hair off the face.

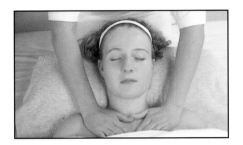

1 *Kneel at the top of your partner's head and lightly oil your palms. With your hands placed over the collarbone, pointing away from you, get ready to begin some gentle* effleurage *strokes.*

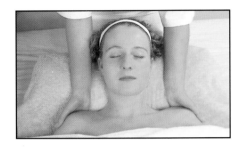

2 *Sweep your hands out across the shoulders, keeping the pressure light.*

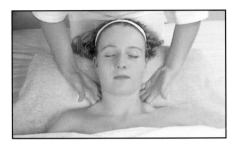

3 *In a continuous movement, bring your hands up round the back of the neck to the nape, pause for a moment, increasing the pressure slightly with the fingertips, then release and lift your hands away.*

Repeat the effleurage *sequence a minimum of three times.*

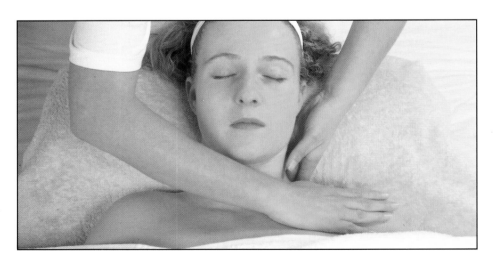

4 *Bring your right arm across the front of your partner so the hand supports the left shoulder. Using light upward strokes, sweep* your left hand up from the top of the shoulder, up the side of the neck to the edge of the jaw. Repeat three times.

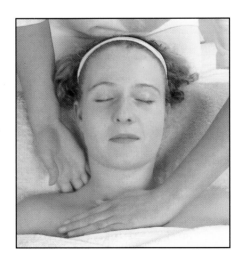

5 *Now repeat this movement on the other side of the neck.*

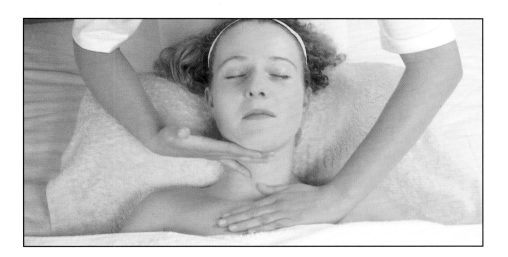

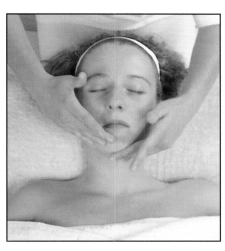

6 *Starting with both hands over the front of the chest, fingers pointing toward each other, lightly sweep the flat of one hand up the front of the neck to the jaw,* *flicking the hand away when you get there. As you flick the first hand away, bring the second up, so you stroke up with alternate hands. Repeat several times.*

7 *Bring both hands up to the front of the jaw. Alternately sweep one hand and then the other up along the jawline toward the ear. Repeat several times.*

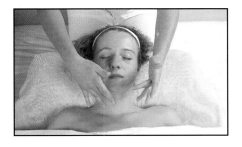

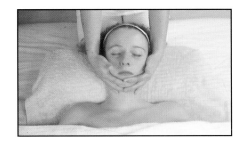

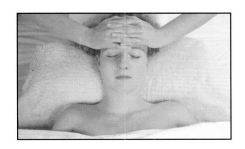

8 *Briskly tap the length of the jawline using the middle and ring fingers, starting from the centre front and working toward the ears. This should be a stimulating movement, so keep the patting quick and fairly firm.*

9 *Afterwards, soothe the area by cradling the face gently with both hands. Pause for several moments then release the hands.*

10 *Bring your hands up to the forehead. Loosely interlock your fingers, and using the palms apply gentle pressure over the forehead. Slowly unlock the fingers to release. Repeat three times.*

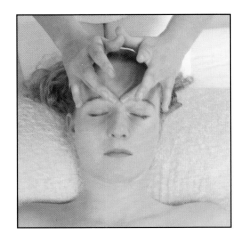

11 *Left: Starting with the third finger of each hand placed on the bridge of the nose, stroke out over the brows toward the temples at each side of the forehead. Come up the forehead a little and, starting again with both fingers at the centre front, repeat the strokes out toward the hairline.*
   Repeat a couple of times more, bringing the fingers higher up the forehead each time, until the whole forehead is covered.

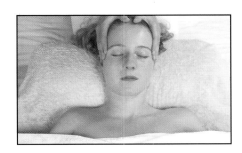

12 *To finish, place your hands on each side of your partner's head, and pause for a few seconds before lifting them away.*

ABDOMEN AND WAIST

Many people feel exposed and vulnerable when baring their abdomen so you will need to be particularly sensitive to your partner when it comes to this part of massage. Start with very gentle strokes, but try to be confident, as a gentle touch which is also tentative can feel unnerving for your partner.

Massage of the abdomen calms the nerves and can soothe stomach aches if they're caused by tension, poor digestion or period pains. It also stimulates the digestive organs so that elimination is improved. You should wait for at least an hour after your partner's meal before giving an abdominal massage.

Kneel beside your partner to do the massage. With a little practice you will find it is possible to tackle both sides from the same position. It helps to start and finish the massage by focusing on your partner's breathing so that your strokes coincide with the intake and expellation. To begin with, try slowly stroking your hands up from the lower abdomen to the chest on inhalation and down the sides on exhalation.

ABDOMEN

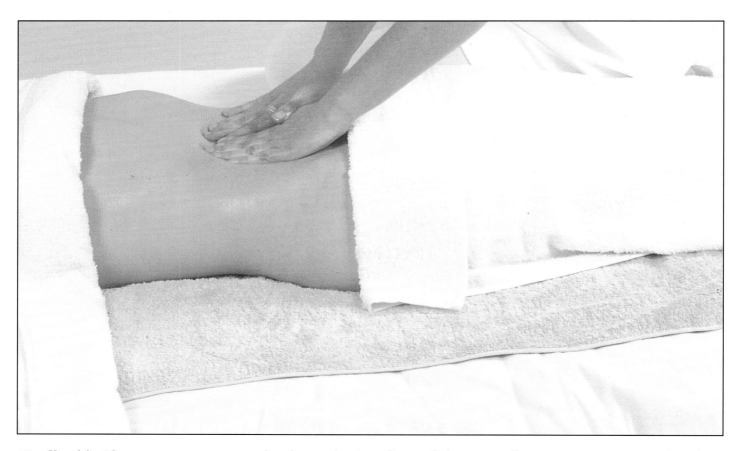

1 *Kneel beside your partner, level with the hips. Lightly oil the palms of the hands, and make contact by gently placing your* hands together in a diamond shape over the lower abdomen, pointing toward the head. Keep the fingers together and the hands relaxed. *Encourage your partner to breathe into the abdomen so you can feel it expand and contract. Work with the breath.*

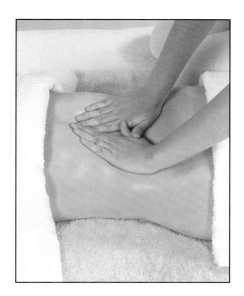

2 *Slowly slide your hands up the centre of the abdomen until you reach the ribs, making sure the pressure is even and not too firm.*

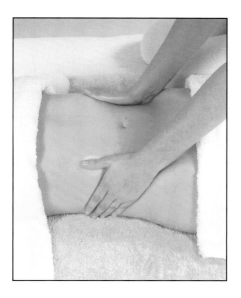

3 *Continue the movement by sweeping the hands out and round the sides of the waist. As you take them out from the ribs toward the sides you can apply a little more pressure, so that you feel the muscles being drawn outward.*

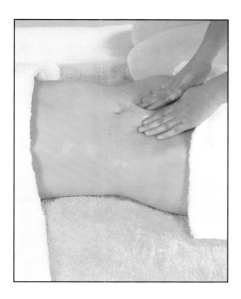

4 *Return to the starting position with both hands placed on the lower abdomen and repeat this continuous movement several times. Apply more oil as necessary.*

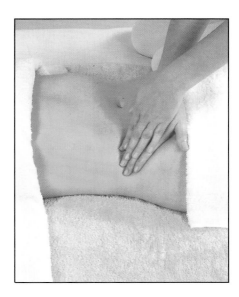

5 *Place both hands on your partner's lower abdomen at the right-hand side, ready to circle the navel. Your left hand rests over the right for support.*

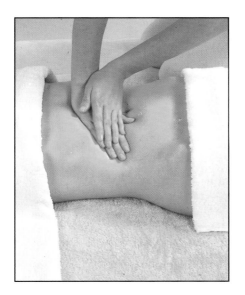

6 *Stroke upward, keeping the left hand over the right, until you reach the ribs. The pressure can be quite firm to stimulate the digestive system. Keep the stroke smooth and continuous.*

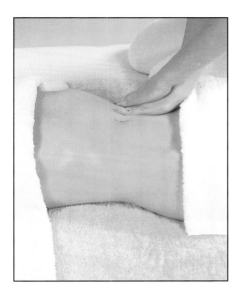

7 *Continue the stroke by bringing your hands across under the ribs, and down the left side of your partner's abdomen. It is important that the direction you work in is up your partner's right side, across and down the left side.*

Repeat the navel-circling movement three times, each time returning to the centre of the lower abdomen.

WAIST

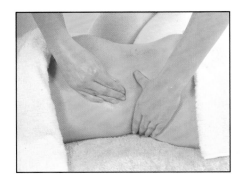

1 *Begin kneading round the waist area by squeezing and releasing the flesh from one hand to the other. These movements should be firm and stimulating.*

2, 3 *Right and below right: Cross your hands over your partner's waist so the palms are grasping the sides of the midriff. Briskly draw them up the side of the waist, uncrossing the hands over the top of the abdomen and turning the palms as they travel down the other side. Draw up again and recross the arms to the original starting position. Keep the speed of this fairly quick and apply firm pressure to draw the flesh up the sides, then lighten your touch across the top of the abdomen. Repeat four times.*

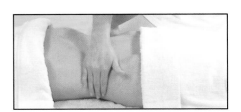

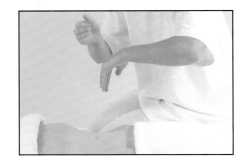

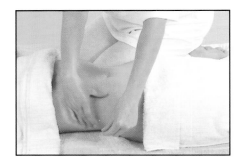

4 *Starting at the far side of the waist, lightly pinch the flesh between fingers and thumbs with brisk, short stimulating movements. Repeat on the other side of the waist.*

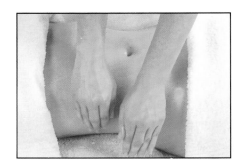

5 *With loosely cupped hands, lightly cup the side of the waist, keeping the pace fast and stimulating, but at the same time checking that it is not causing discomfort. The action should be enough to increase the flow of blood to the area without hurting.*

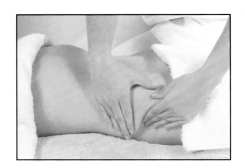

6 *Working on the top of the hip area, squeeze and release the flesh in a kneading movement, using deep and stimulating pressure.*

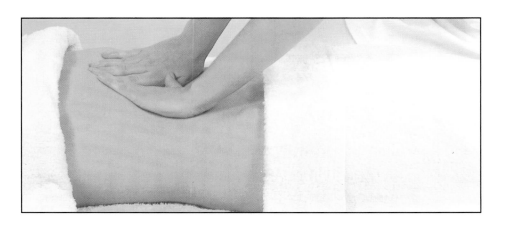

7 *Left: Finish the massage of the abdomen by repeating the soothing effleurage strokes from the beginning of the sequence. End with both hands placed over the centre of the abdomen, fingers pointing toward the head. Hold for a few seconds before lifting off.*

BACK OF BODY

*Ask your partner to turn over on to their front, ready for you to start work
on the back of the legs and buttocks. Rest their head to one side.*

LEGS AND BUTTOCKS

*The backs of the legs and buttocks offer plenty of scope
for massage techniques. Most people can take plenty of
firm massage on the larger muscles in the thighs and
buttocks. The fleshy parts are ideal for kneading and
squeezing and the firmer pressure can feel wonderfully
satisfying. In contrast though, the most gentle effleurage
can still stimulate other body functions to improve their
efficiency. Poor circulation and a sluggish lymphatic
system can be considerably improved with a good leg
massage. Tiredness and heaviness in the legs is
alleviated and your partner should have a renewed
feeling of energy afterwards.*

EFFLEURAGE

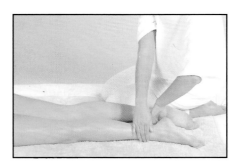

1 *Left: Start by kneeling on one
side of your partner's ankles.
You should be able to work on both
legs from the same side. Begin by
working on the leg furthest away
from you.*
   *Lightly oil your hands and place
them crossed over the back of the
left ankle.*

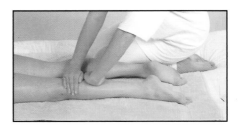 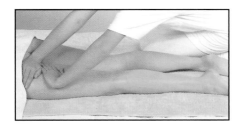 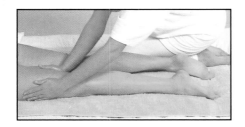

2 *In a smooth and continuous
movement, effleurage up the
leg, with right hand leading the
left. When you get to the back of
the knee pause for two seconds.*

3 *Carry the stroke up the leg and
at the top of the thigh cross
the hands, keeping the pressure
even and light.*

4 *Bring your hands back down
the sides of the leg until you
reach the back of the ankle again.*

*Repeat the sequence three times, each time increasing the pressure slightly
on the upward stroke toward the heart.*

UPPER LEGS AND BUTTOCKS

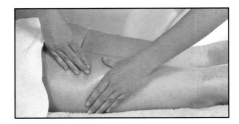

1 *Move to a kneeling position beside your partner's upper leg. Using a firm kneading movement, squeeze and release the back of the thigh muscles, working up to the buttocks. You should be able to pick up quite a large area of muscle between the hands.*

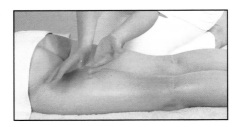

2 *With the outside edge of the hands, do some short sharp hacking movements. Alternate the hands in a quick, repetitive action. Continue the hacking all over the back of the upper leg and the buttocks.*

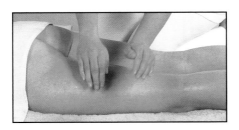

3 *Continue working on the upper leg and buttocks, with some cupping. The cupping action should be short and fast to stimulate the whole area.*

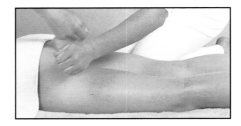

4 *With loose fists, briskly pound the top and outside of the thigh. You can use the backs of your fingers or the outside edge of the fists. Use a firmer knuckling action over the buttock area.*

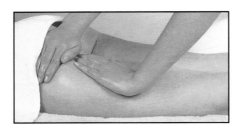

5 *Follow this sequence of friction movements with soothing* effleurage *strokes from the back of the knee to the top of the thigh, sweeping out and back down the leg to the knee.*

CALVES

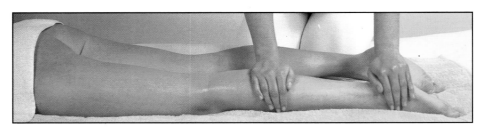

1 *Move back down to kneel beside your partner's ankles. Lightly oil your hands again if necessary. Start with both hands on the back of your partner's ankle. Smooth your right hand up toward the knee, keeping your left hand on the ankle for support.*

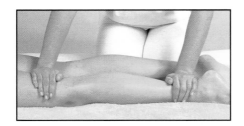

2 *Continue to stroke the right hand toward the thigh, keeping the pressure light as you reach the back of the knee.*

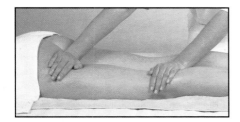

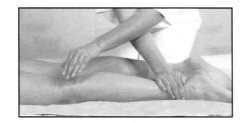

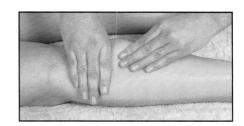

3 *As you continue the stroke, taking your right hand up toward the top of the thigh, simultaneously slide your left hand up the lower leg to the back of the knee. Try to make this a flowing movement.*

4 *Without pausing, bring your right hand in a continuous stroke back down the leg. When you reach the knee you will need to slide the left hand off the knee, so the right hand can continue right down to the ankle again.*

5 *Start kneading the calf with both hands, working from the ankle up to the knee. Don't knead the back of the knee. Squeeze and release the calf muscle as you go. If your partner's calf muscles are particularly tight this kneading action may feel uncomfortable, so ask your partner if the pressure is right.*

Repeat three times, or until you feel confident with the movement.

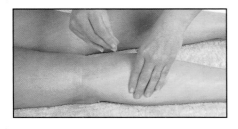

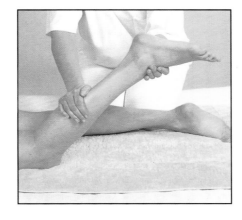

6 *Do some short, sharp pinching movements all over the calf muscle, again checking that you are not hurting your partner.*

7 *Left: Lifting and supporting your partner's leg in the left hand, slide your right hand up from the back of the ankle to the knee. Keep the pressure as firm as is comfortable. Repeat three times. Gently return the leg to rest on the floor.*

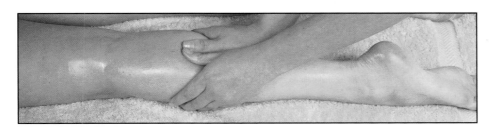

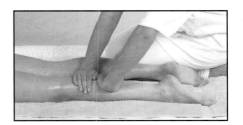

8 *With your thumbs together start at the back of the ankle, and work up the back of the calf to the knee, applying pressure firm enough to release tightness in these* muscles. *When you reach the back of the knee, lighten the pressure and sweep your hands back down the sides of the leg to the ankle. Repeat three times.*

9 *To complete the back of the leg massage, repeat the* effleurage *strokes from the beginning of the sequence, stroking the leg from ankle to thigh and back down to the ankle again. Repeat three times to soothe the leg.*

Repeat the entire back of leg massage on your partner's other leg, covering the leg you have worked on with a towel to keep the muscles warm.

BACK AND SHOULDERS

The back is an area of great strength and mobility, and it is the main supportive structure of the body. It therefore warrants more attention than most other areas. By working on the back you can reach nerves affecting every part of the body.

Full back massage, with emphasis on the spine and lower back, greatly alleviates effects of stress throughout the body, enhancing physical and psychological well-being. Smooth, flowing strokes stretch the muscles and tissues round contours of the back, and help restore flexibility for health and mobility, whilst stronger strokes along the spinal muscles and over the lower back bring deeper relief to aching or knotted muscles.

You should never massage directly on the spine itself, although working down each side is highly beneficial. Avoid using percussion strokes such as hacking and cupping on the kidneys, which are level with the waistline in the centre of the back.

First, make sure your partner is comfortable, lying face down with arms resting beside the face. Support the forehead with a rolled towel, and if helpful, use a pillow, cushion or rolled towel under the chest. It helps to have hair clear from the back of the neck.

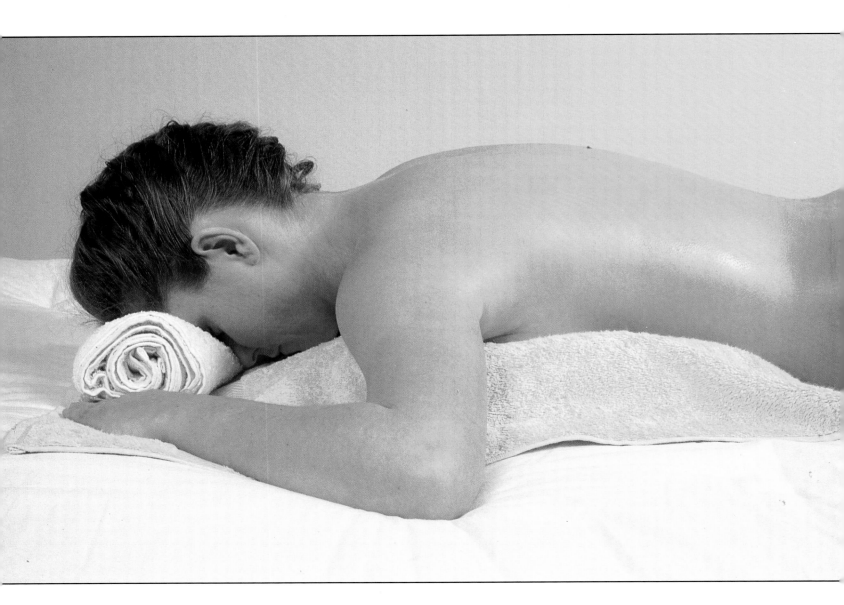

EFFLEURAGE

Kneel beside your partner's right hip and oil your hands. With your first long effleurage *strokes try to concentrate on finding areas of particular tension and tightness.*

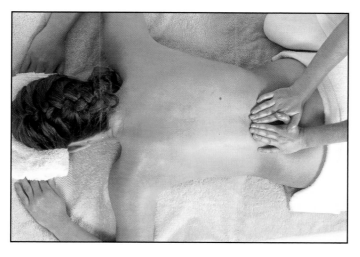

1 *Starting at the lower back begin the* effleurage *strokes. With thumbs crossed to connect the hands together, move slowly up the centre of the back, putting firm pressure on the fingertips.*

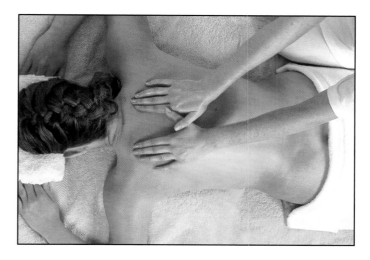

2 *Take the stroke up to the top of the back in a continuous movement.*

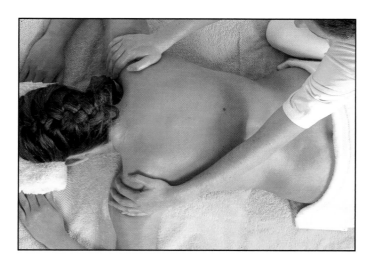

3 *Without a pause, separate the hands at the top of the back, sweeping them out and round the shoulders.*

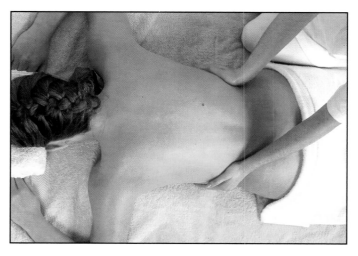

4 *Continue the stroke, bringing both hands down the sides of the back to the lower back, ready to begin again.*

Repeat this effleurage *sequence three times, oiling your hands each time.*

SHOULDERS

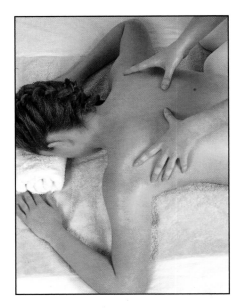

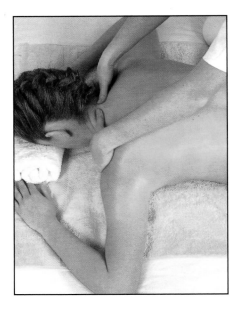

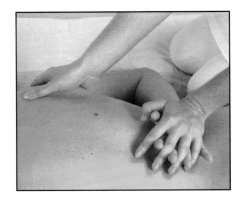

1 *Using your thumbs each side of the spine, start level with the shoulder blades and make circling pressure movements, working quite firmly into the muscles.*

2 *Continue working up each side of the spine until you reach the nape of the neck.*

3 *Carefully bring your partner's arm across the hollow of the back and clasp their right hand with your left to support the arm. The shoulder blade should now stick out slightly. With your right thumb make circular pressure movements over the shoulder area. Strong muscles support the shoulder blade and you can work firmly under the bone itself to release tightness in this area.*

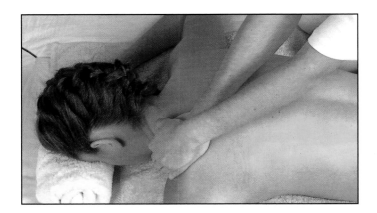

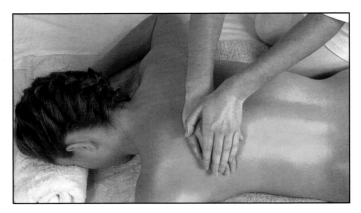

4 *With your left hand resting over your right to increase the pressure, work in small, circular movements from the base of the neck out over the shoulder.*

5 *Continue round to the shoulder blade, using firm pressure to release tension in the muscle.*

Move to the other side of your partner and repeat these steps on the other shoulder.

BACK

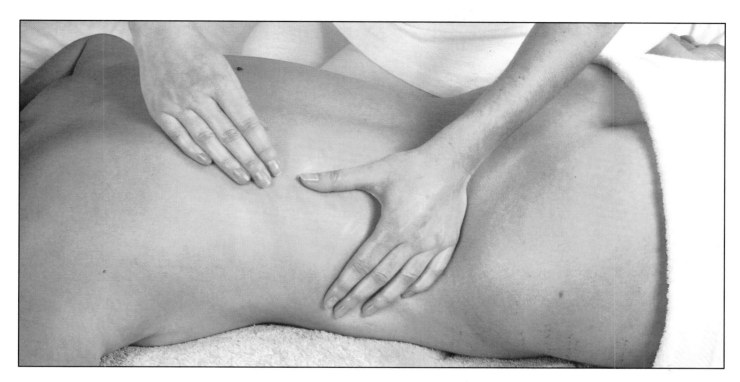

1 *Kneeling to the right side of your partner, start to knead the far side of the back firmly with both hands, beginning at the outer* sides of the waist. Pick up, roll and release the muscles, alternately pressing one hand toward another. Continue kneading up the back *until you reach the shoulders. Start again at the waist but this time come closer to the spine and repeat the line of kneading up the back.*

Repeat the kneading on the near side of the back. You should be able to do this without moving your kneeling position.

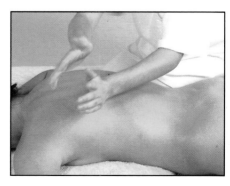

2 *Using the outer edge of the hands, briskly and rhythmically hack from the lower back up to the shoulders, but avoid the bony shoulder blade. Try to visualize each side of the back divided into three sections, so you cover the whole back thoroughly.*

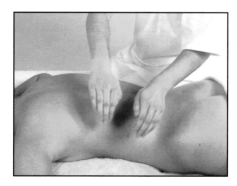

3 *Start cupping from the lower back up the back and across the shoulders. The action should be quick, with alternate hands striking the back briskly.*

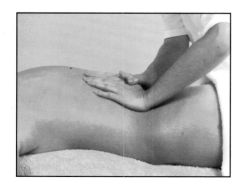

4 *Repeat the* effleurage *strokes from the beginning of the sequence to soothe the back. Repeat a number of times.*

SPINE

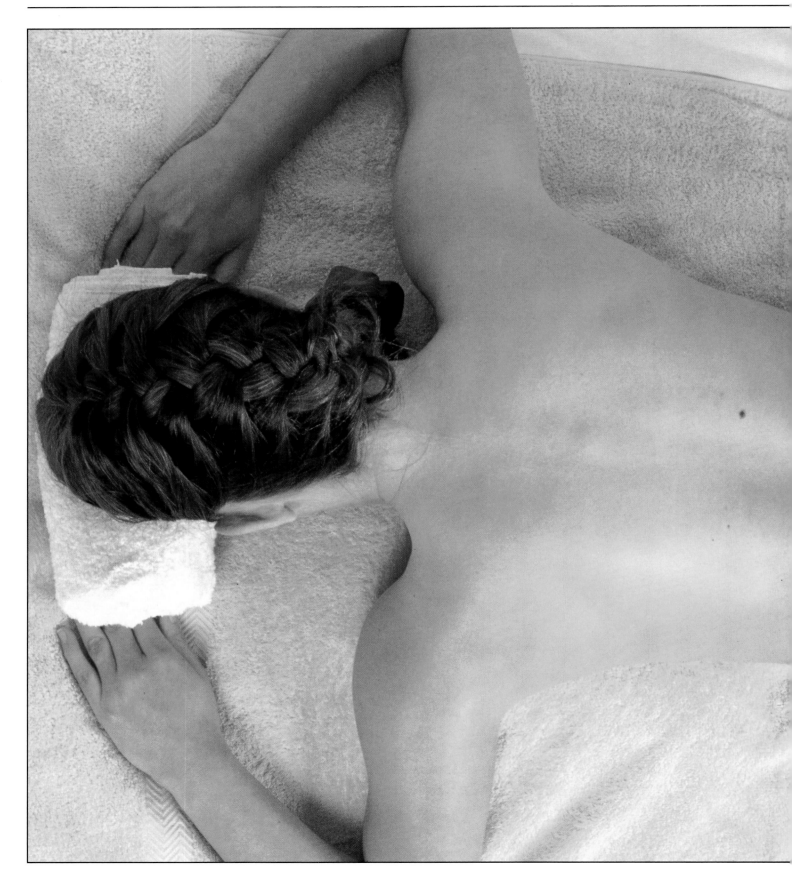

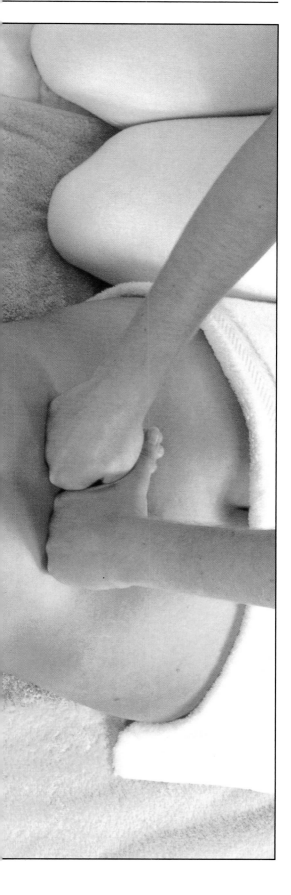

1 *Left: With loose fists, and thumbs crossed for support, push the top of the hands up each side of the spine to the nape of the neck.*

2 *Right: Uncurl the fingers when you get to the nape and sweep them back down the sides of the back. Repeat three times.*

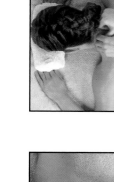

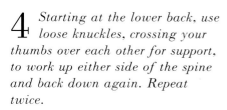

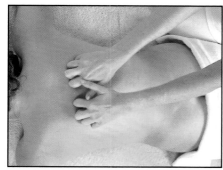

3 *Starting at the lower back, place the thumbs on either side of the spine, resting your hands either side of the back. Rotate the thumbs in small circles, travelling up the sides of the spine until you reach the hairline. Use firm pressure. Reverse the movement, circling your thumbs back down each side of the spine.*

4 *Starting at the lower back, use loose knuckles, crossing your thumbs over each other for support, to work up either side of the spine and back down again. Repeat twice.*

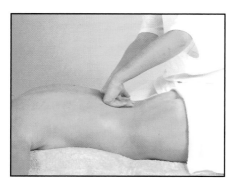

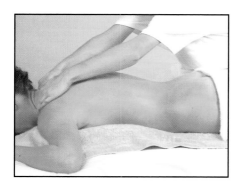

5 *Using the backs of your hands and starting at the lower back, push up either side of the spine to just above the waistline. Then sweep your hands outward and back down round the hips. Repeat three times.*

6 *To finish the massage, repeat the effleurage strokes from the beginning of the sequence, starting at the lower back, up the back, round the shoulders and down again to the lower back, in a continuous sweeping movement.*

SELF MASSAGE

A simple, effective self massage can do wonders to ease away tension and restore energy after a stressful, tiring day. After a shower or bath, massaging the body with lotions and oils is very relaxing and helps keep the skin in glowing condition.

You can use self massage to target particular aches and pains or areas of tension, for relief just where you need it. The beauty of self massage is you can do it to suit your needs and moods at any time – to unwind in the evening or to energize yourself in the morning.

SHOULDERS

1 *Sitting upright, start from the base of the neck and press down with your fingers along the top of the shoulders. As you reach the bony part of the shoulder, slide your hand back to the base of the neck, and repeat the pressing at least three times. Finish by stroking firmly from neck to shoulder and then repeat on the other side of the neck.*

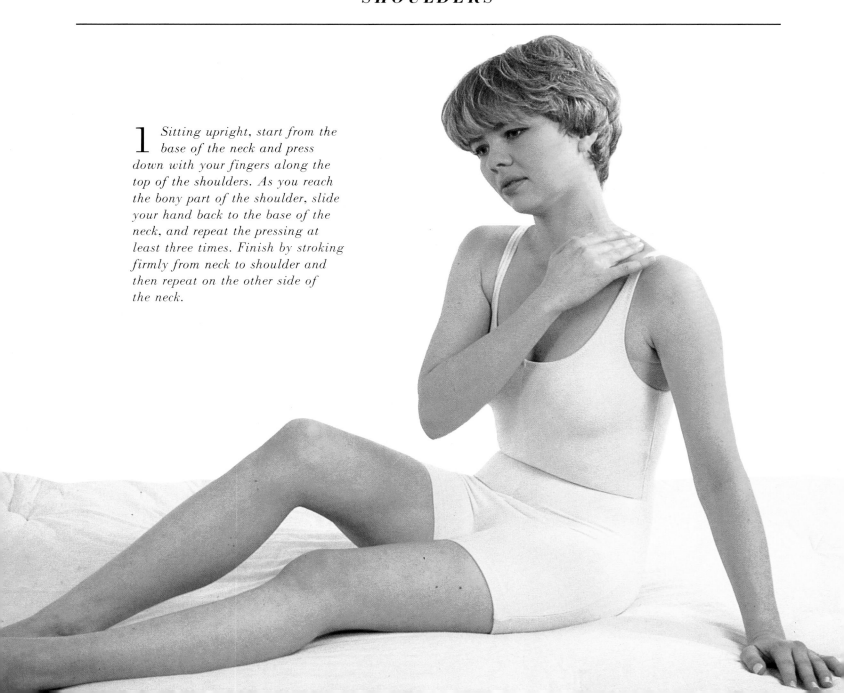

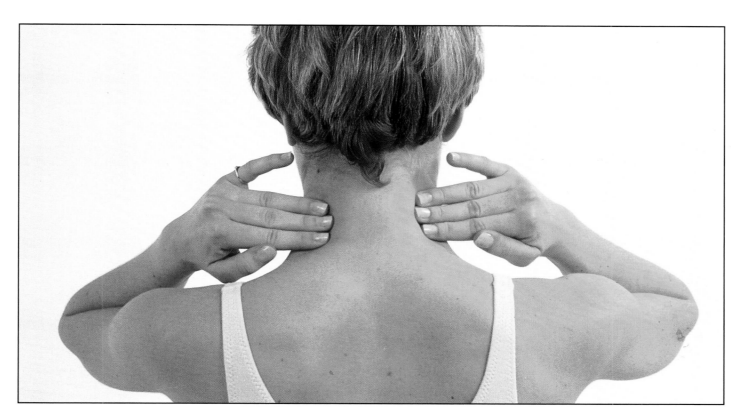

2 *Use the fingertips of both hands to make small circular movements, working up the back of the neck. Gentle circular movements, where you can feel yourself easing muscular tightness, are better than direct, static pressures on this area. Continue up and round the base of the skull.*

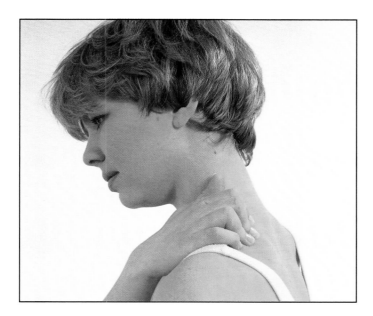

3 *Knead each shoulder with a firm squeezing action, rolling the flesh between your fingers and the ball of the hand. Repeat several times on each side.*

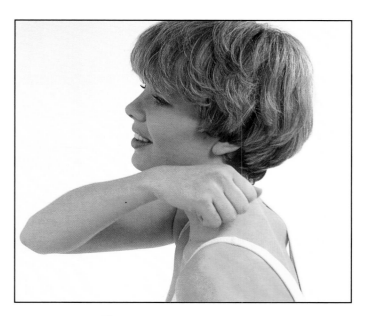

4 *With your hand in a loose fist, pummel your shoulder lightly, keeping the wrist and elbow relaxed. Use light, springy movements to stimulate the area. Repeat on the other shoulder.*

ARMS

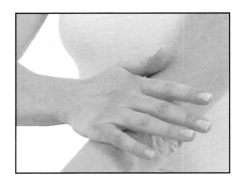

1 Stroke firmly up the arm from the wrist to the shoulder, returning with a lighter touch. Repeat the stroke several times on different parts of the arm.

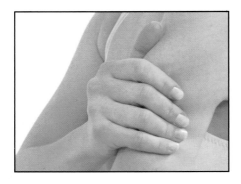

2 Pressing your fingers toward the palm of the hand, knead up the arm from the elbow to the shoulder. Cover the area thoroughly, working right round the arm.

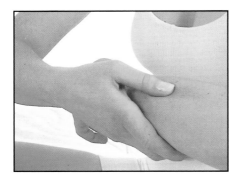

3 Starting from the wrist, knead up the forearm toward the elbow, this time using your thumb to make circular movements.

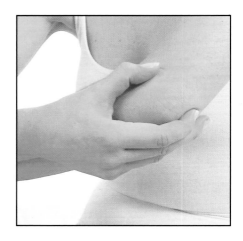

4 With thumb and fingers make circular pressures round the elbow. First, work round the far side of the elbow with your working arm coming over the top of the arm you're massaging, then bend that arm up and work from the inside of your elbow. You may need more oil for dry elbows.

5 Right: Gently but briskly pat your upper arm, or use some gentle cupping. Follow with some effleurage stroking up and down the whole arm again to finish. Work on the hand before massaging the other arm.

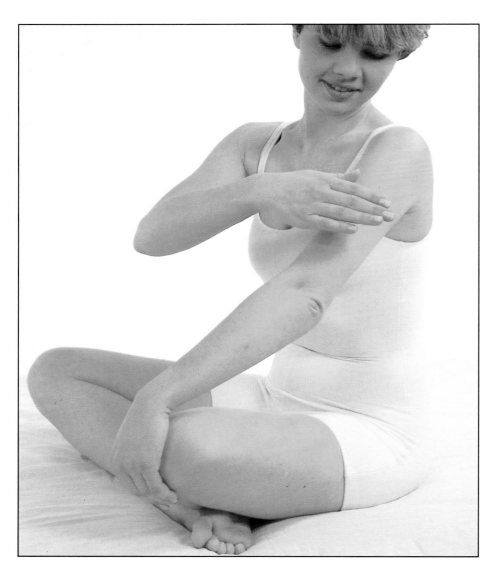

HANDS

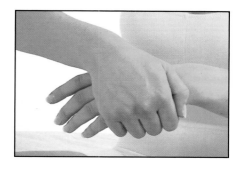 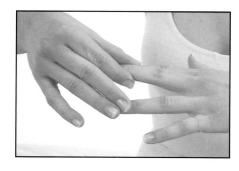 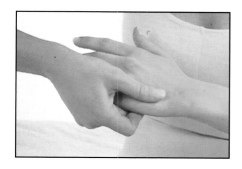

1 *Squeeze the hand firmly, spreading the palm laterally. Cover the whole of the hand, fingers and wrist.*

2 *Using circular pressure, squeeze each finger joint between your finger and thumb. Then hold the base of each finger and pull the finger gently to stretch it, sliding your grip up to the top of the finger in a continuous movement.*

3 *With circular thumb pressures, work up each of the furrows between the bones in the hand, from the knuckle to the wrist. When you have covered each furrow, smooth the hand by stroking.*

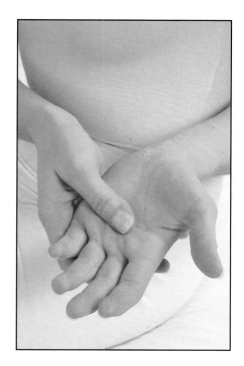 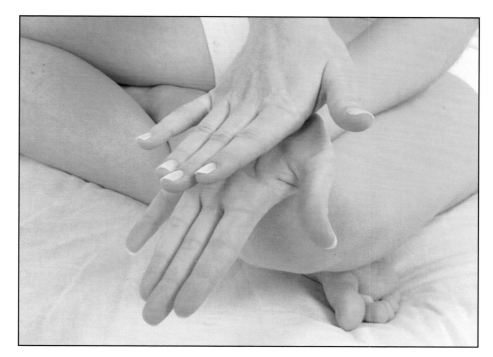

4 *Turn the hand over to work on the palm. Cover the area with circular thumb pressures, paying particular attention to the heel of the hand and the wrist. Follow this with some deeper, static pressures all over the palm.*

5 *Finish by stroking the palm of one hand with the other. This can be quite a firm stroke, working from the tips of the fingers to the wrist, leading with the pressure*

from the heel of the hand. Stroke back to the fingers and repeat twice more, each time using slightly less pressure. Finally, stroke the inside of the wrist.

Repeat the whole of the arm and hand massage sequences on the other side.

BACK AND ABDOMEN

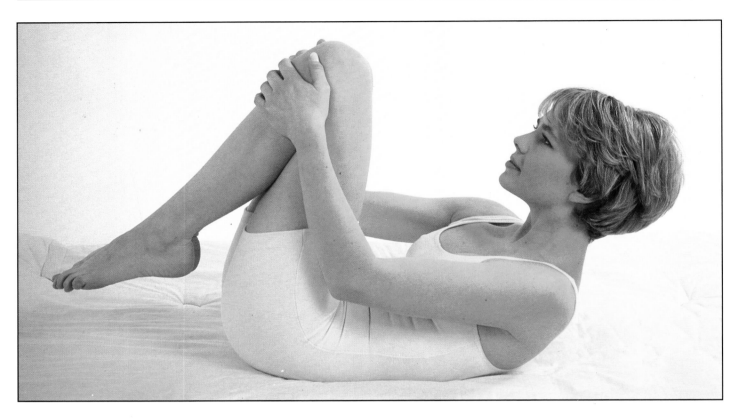

1 *Lie on your back, clasp your knees and gently rock backward and forward to massage the lower back, buttocks and hip joints and gently stretch out the vertebrae.*

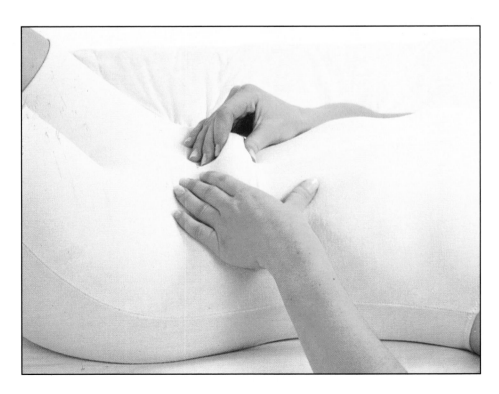

2 *Left: Bend your knees up and use some gentle petrissage to knead the whole of the abdominal area. When you have finished kneading, place both hands flat on the centre of the abdomen, fingers pointing slightly together, and pause for a few moments. Then smooth your hands outward over the hips and thighs in a long, slow, moulding movement.*

BUTTOCKS, HIPS AND THIGHS

1 *Kneel up and pummel your hips and buttocks, using a clenched fist and keeping your wrists flexible.*

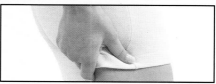

2 *With the thumb and fingers, squeeze and release the muscles firmly and slowly, working from the top of the thigh over the buttock. Repeat on the left side.*

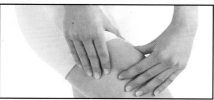

3 *Use both hands to squeeze and release the muscles on the front and side of the thigh, kneading the entire upper leg. Repeat on the other side.*

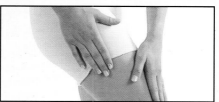

4 *Starting at the knee, stroke up the thigh with both hands to soothe the leg.*

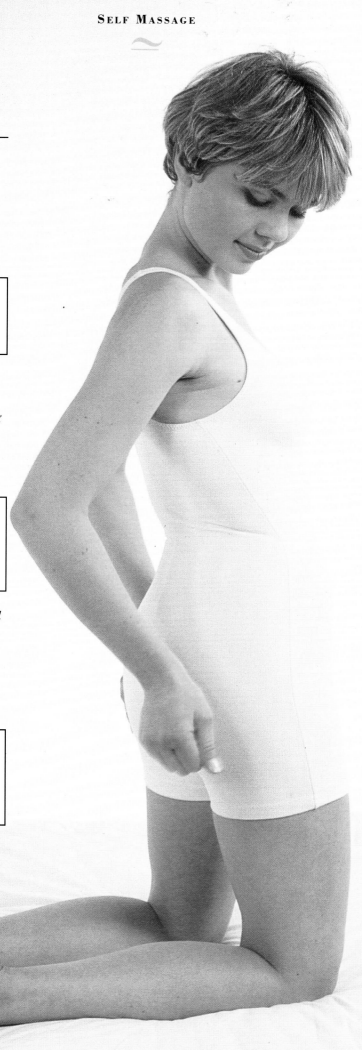

LEGS

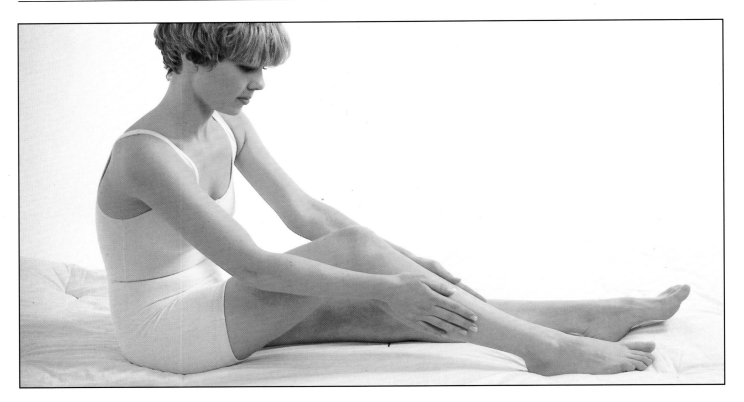

1 Sitting down, with one leg raised slightly, stroke the leg with both hands from ankle to thigh. Begin the stroke as close to the ankle as you can reach. Repeat several times, moving round the leg slightly each time to stroke a different part.

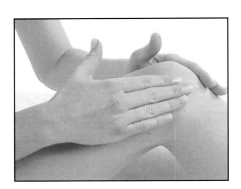

2 Massage the knee, stroking round the outside of the kneecap to begin with, then using circular pressure with the fingertips to work round the kneecap more firmly.

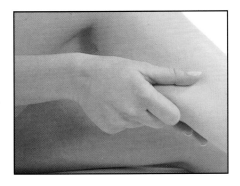

3 Knead the calf muscle with both hands, using a firm petrissage to loosen any tension in the muscle.

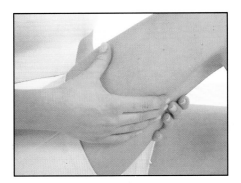

4 Continue the kneading on the thigh, working over the top and outside areas with alternate hands. Whilst the leg is still raised, do some soothing effleurage strokes up the back of the leg from ankle to hip.

Continue with the foot massage (opposite) before repeating all the steps on the other leg.

FEET

1 *Sitting down and leaning back, raise a leg, supporting the weight with your hands. Rotate the right ankle five times in each direction.*

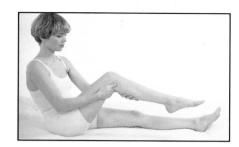

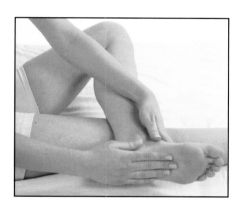

2 *Gently bring your foot over the other leg. With one hand on top of the foot and one underneath, stroke up the foot from toes to ankle. Repeat three times.*

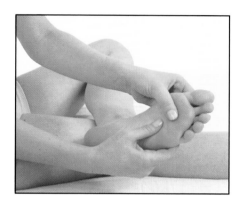

3 *With the thumbs, apply circular pressure over the ball of the foot. Work in lines from the inside of the foot to the outer edge. Repeat three times.*

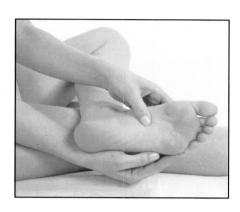

4 *Supporting the foot with one hand, continue the circular pressures over the raised instep, working from the inner to the outer edge. Repeat three times.*

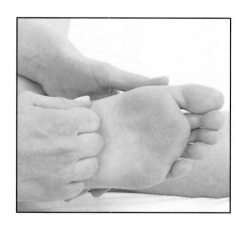

5 *Still holding the foot with one hand, make a loose fist with the other and firmly rotate your fist over the instep. Work thoroughly into the arch.*

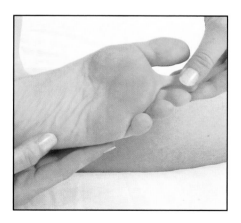

6 *Massage each toe individually. Slowly stretch the toe between the thumb and finger, pull gently, moving your fingers up the toe each time, until you reach the tip.*

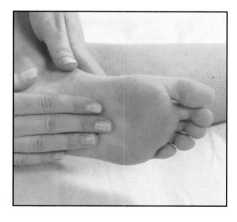

7 *Repeat the effleurage strokes of the foot, with one hand over and one under the foot, working from toes to ankle, several times.*

Repeat the leg and foot massage sequence on the other side.

MASSAGE AND EXERCISE

Professional sports people value massage very highly, not least because it works on several levels. Used before exercise it can prepare the body for the increase in activity not only by warming and loosening the muscles and joints (increasing their flexibility and helping to prevent cramp and injuries), but also by stimulating the system, both physically and mentally. This is the key to improved performance. After an exercise session, massage speeds up the elimination of waste products (in particular lactic acid) by stimulating the lymphatic system. The accumulation of these waste products during exercise is the cause of much of the stiffness and pain experienced afterwards.

STRAINS AND SPRAINS

A burning sensation under the skin is likely to indicate that muscles, fibres or ligaments have been strained – stretched beyond their natural limits. This is often the result of exercising without an adequate warm-up routine or over-exertion. A routine of pre-exercise massage and limbering will help to prevent strains. Gently massaging the affected area will also help to speed recovery.

Sprains are more serious and are caused by violent wrenching of a joint, most commonly the ankle, wrist or knee. The surrounding muscles, ligaments and tendons may also be damaged and the affected area may be extremely painful and swollen. Apply an ice-pack or cold compress for 15–20 minutes to reduce the swelling. When it is removed you can start to massage the area gently (as shown opposite), taking care not to work directly on the swelling. Rest the ankle as much as possible and use a support bandage.

A serious sprain should always be checked by a doctor in case a bone has been fractured, and a sprained knee always requires medical attention.

CRAMP

You don't have to be a fitness fanatic to suffer from cramp. On the contrary, it is usually underused or ill-prepared muscles which go into cramp. It doesn't even take movement to set it off: the searing pain of cramp can occur in the middle of the night, when the reduced circulation has caused muscles to contract. Frequent cramps may indicate generally poor circulation or a deficiency of calcium or salt. Massage will increase the blood circulation to alleviate the pain. You should also try to stretch out the affected muscle.

BACKACHE

Back strain is the most common source of debilitating pain. Most sports put increased strain on the legs, buttocks and back. Previous injuries can make the back prone to recurrent pain. Awkward, inappropriate or excessive exercise can also cause trouble. You should never subject the back to unnecessary strain. With regular and thorough back massage (particularly before exercise) the likelihood of injury is reduced. If, however, you want a quick warm-up for the back, or an after-exercise sequence, follow the instant back and shoulder massage. Always consult a doctor, osteopath or chiropractor if in any doubt about the seriousness of a back problem.

WITH OR WITHOUT OILS

You don't always have oil at hand, and it certainly isn't crucial for massaging unexpected strains, sprains and cramps. If you do have some light vegetable oil nearby, all the better, but don't worry if you don't.

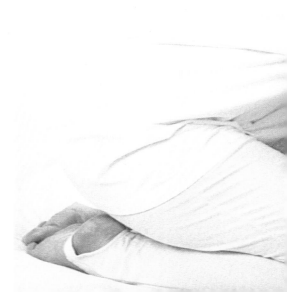

ANKLE STRAIN OR SPRAIN

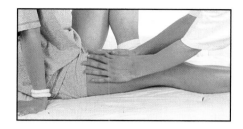

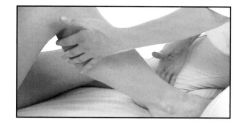

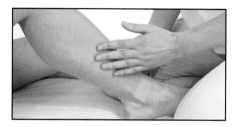

1 *Above and below: Avoid working directly on the swollen area. Start with gentle effleurage strokes working from the knee toward the thigh. Massaging in the direction of the lymph nodes in the groin will help drain away the fluids that have accumulated round the joint. Lightly stroke back to the knee. Repeat several times.*

2 *Help your partner to bend the affected leg. Continue the effleurage strokes on the lower leg, this time working from the ankle to the knee, alternating your hands. Repeat several times, then gently squeeze the calves with one hand, with the other supporting the foot.*

3 *Concentrating on the ankle area, stroke extremely gently all round the ankle with short upward movements. Check that this is not causing discomfort.*

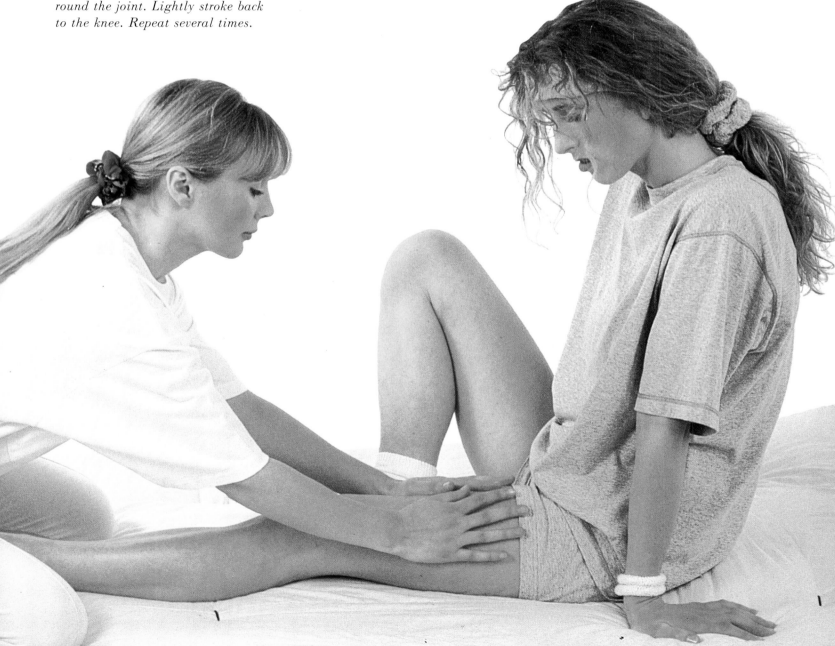

CALF CRAMP

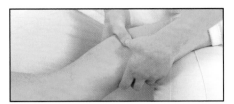

1 With your partner lying face
down and the foot supported
across your leg or a small pillow,
gradually apply direct thumb
pressure into the belly of the
cramped calf muscle for eight to ten
seconds.

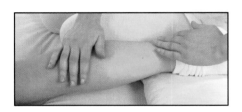

2 Do some effleurage strokes,
working from ankle to thigh
and back down again.

SELF-HELP STRETCH

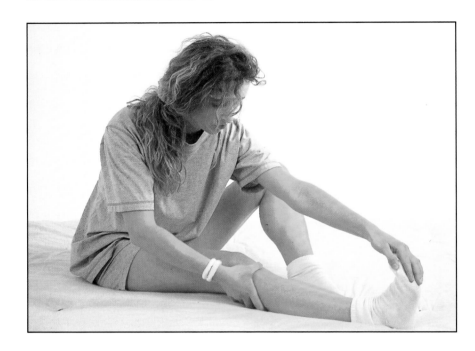

A good way of dealing with calf
cramp is to sit down with the
affected leg straight and stretch
the toes toward you. Hold this
position for eight seconds and
then release. Repeat a few times,
until the spasm seems to be
lessening. Then knead your calf
muscle using firm pressure.
When the muscle feels more
relaxed switch to effleurage
strokes, working up the leg.

HAMSTRING CRAMP

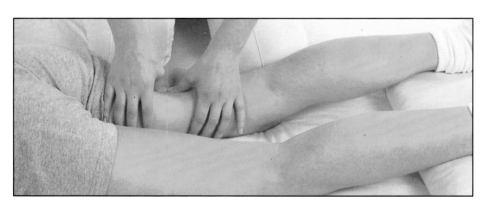

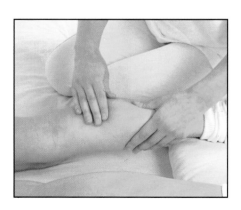

1 With your partner lying face
down and the ankles raised on
a small pillow or cushion, begin
massaging up the back of the thigh
using alternate hands in slow,
rhythmical stroking movements.
Then apply static pressure to the
middle of the thigh with the
thumbs, holding for eight to ten
seconds.

2 Firmly knead the calf muscle.
Squeeze, press and release the
muscle using one hand after the
other. Finally, do some soothing
effleurage strokes up from ankle to
thigh and back down again.

HAMSTRING SELF-HELP STRETCH

Lie down flat, with the affected leg raised and the other knee bent. Stretch the muscle by pulling the thigh gently toward the chest.

Then firmly stroke up the back of your thigh for eight to ten seconds. Start to knead the back of the thigh until you feel the muscles begin to relax. Finally stroke over the area to soothe it.

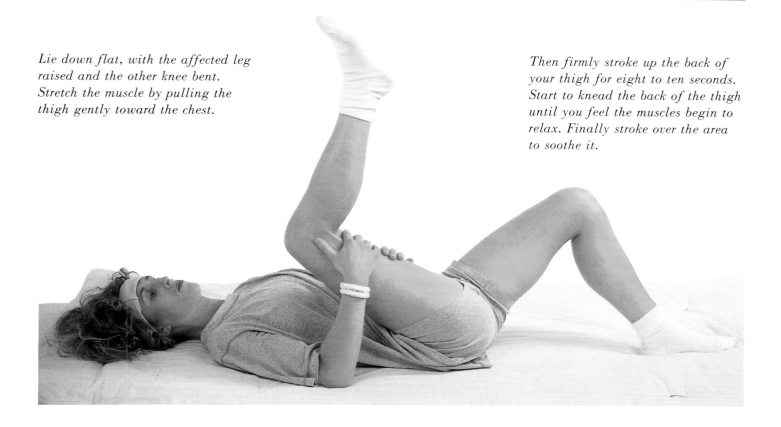

TENNIS OR GOLFER'S ELBOW

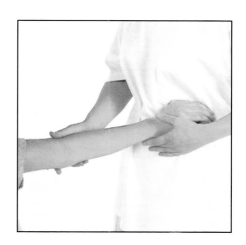

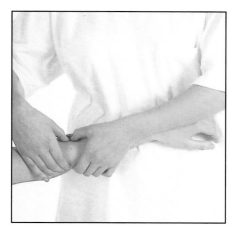

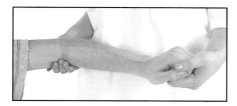

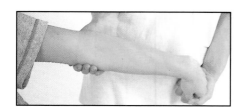

1 Support your partner's wrist in one hand and use soothing effleurage strokes along both sides of the arm, stroking from the wrist to the elbow and back again. Repeat several times.

2 Rest your partner's hand against your side. Continue working up from the wrist to the elbow and back, making small circular movements with both thumbs, paying particular attention to the muscles in the forearm.

3,4 Secure your partner's hand in yours, and with the other hand supporting the elbow, flex the elbow forward, bringing the hand back to give the tendons that attach to the bones a good stretch.

BABY MASSAGE

A newborn baby instinctively responds to touch, and massage between mother and baby is a marvellous way of enhancing the natural bonding. All babies have this powerful sensitivity to being caressed and cuddled. Watch how a baby tightly curls its hands or toes as soon as something touches them.

There is no fixed sequence for massaging a baby. Keep the movements gentle and flowing. The simple action of gently stroking a baby will strengthen the natural bonding, and soothe and reassure the baby too. Massage has been shown to help calm difficult or colicky babies, and alleviate wind and other digestive problems. It may also build resistence to coughs and colds. Use a little light vegetable oil which is easily absorbed, such as sweet almond or sunflower, taking care to avoid the eyes.

GETTING COMFORTABLE

Lay the baby gently on the back on a warm, soft towel between your legs, or on your lap, whichever is most comfortable. Pour about 1 teaspoon (5 ml) of sweet almond oil into a small dish. Make sure your hands are warm and that the room is quiet, very warm and there are no draughts. After a baby's bathtime is ideal.

WORKING ON BABY'S FRONT

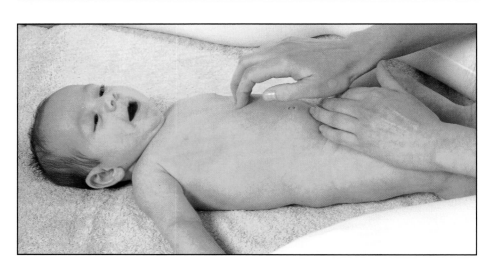

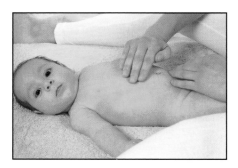

1 *Slowly and gently, smooth a little of the oil all over the front of the baby's body, shoulders to feet, avoiding the face. Lightly* stroke down the chest and abdomen, with the tips of your fingers. This is a delightful stroke which can be used to calm a baby anytime.

2 *Keeping the pressure very light, smooth both hands over the abdomen in continuous circular strokes, working up the baby's right side, across and down the baby's left side. Keep the movement continuous by lifting your left hand when your arms cross. Repeat these circular strokes several times.*

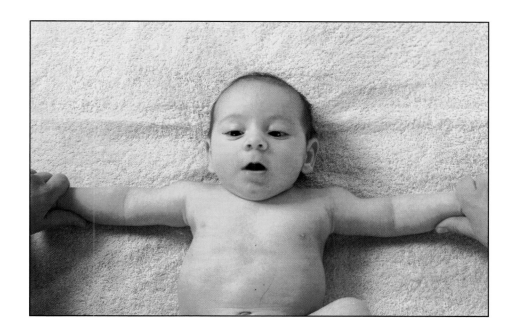

3 *Left: Gently stretch out both arms to the side, spreading the hands and fingers if the baby will let you. Gently squeeze out along the arms, then massage the wrist and palms with light, circular thumb movements. Finish by stretching out each finger with a slight pull.*

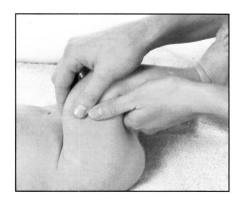

4 *Move on to the legs and feet, working on one leg at a time. Support the leg with both hands and gently squeeze and release the fleshy part of the thigh. Then, supporting the leg with one hand, stroke the leg from the knee to the thigh and back down again.*

5 *Right: Move your supporting hand down to behind the ankle. Gently smooth the palm of your other hand over the top of the foot from toe to ankle and back again. When you get to the toes, very gently stretch each one in turn.*

Repeat steps 4 and 5 on the baby's other leg.

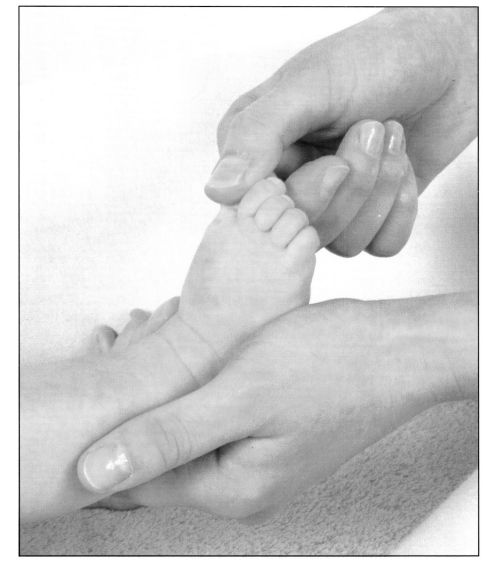

WORKING ON BABY'S BACK

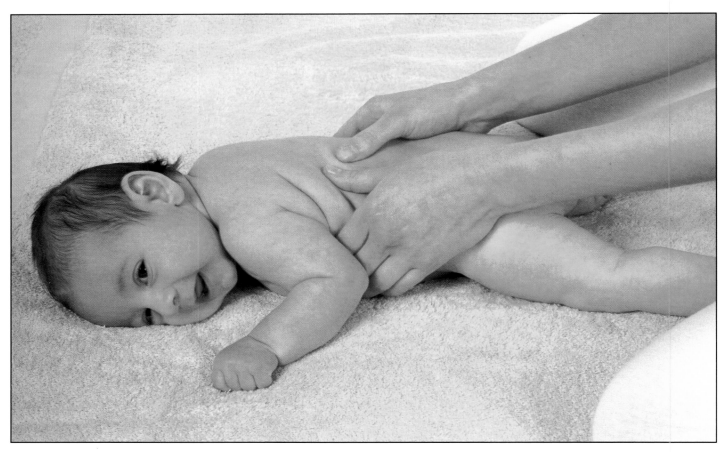

1 *Turn the baby over on to the front. Begin by stroking up the whole back to distribute a little oil.*

Take your strokes round the sides as well and then up the legs, back and out over the arms. Gentle

massage on the back like this is particularly soothing because of its calming effect on the spinal nerves.

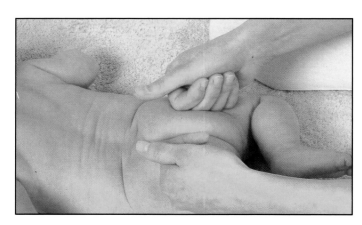

2 *Gently knead and squeeze the buttocks to stimulate the circulation. Make a loose fist and rotate over the buttocks, in circular movements.*

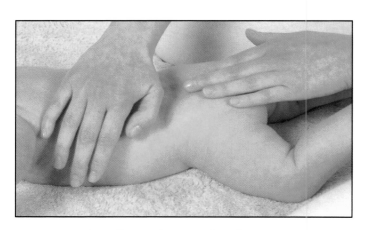

3 *Alternating your hands, one over the other, gently stroke up one side of the back to the shoulders and down again. Repeat on the other side of the back.*

4 *Bring both hands round the sides of the upper body, and use your thumbs to massage gently up the back to the base of the neck, and down again. Include some gentle massage with the thumbs on the shoulders.*

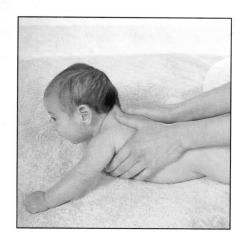

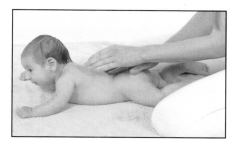

5 *To finish, repeat the feather strokes used at the beginning of the massage, working all over the back from neck to buttocks.*

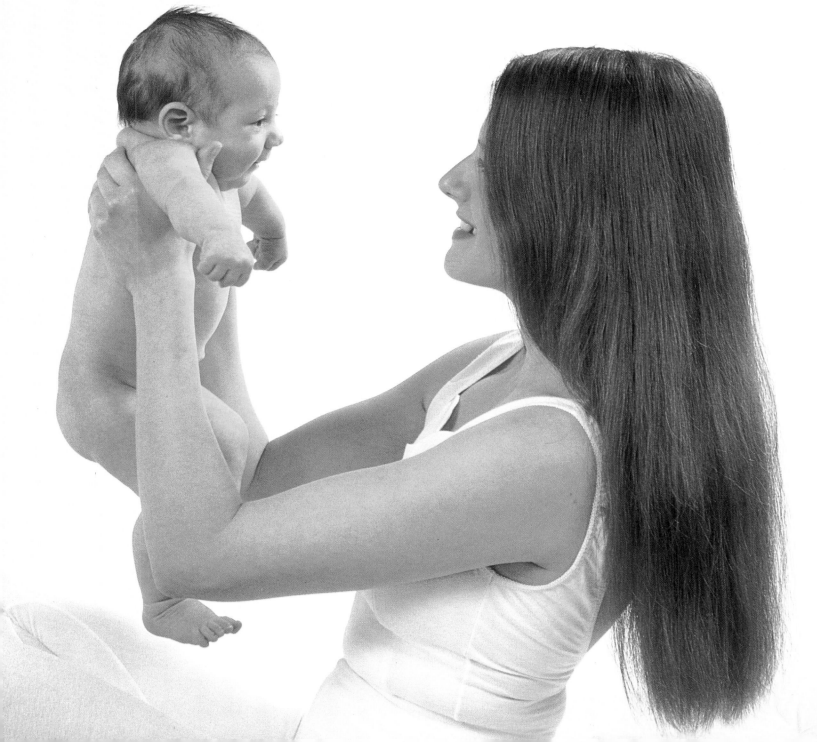

MASSAGE FOR OLDER PEOPLE

As we get older, painful, stiff joints, rheumatism and other signs of wear and tear become all too common. There are many ways to minimize the discomfort that the aging process brings. Good nutrition and remaining as active as possible are as crucial as ever, and massage can help in reducing pain, alleviating stiffness and retaining mobility. Increasing the blood circulation and gently releasing stiffness and inflexibility, it is a good way to help keep active. It isn't necessary to lie down – sitting on a chair is fine for massage of the neck and shoulders, and you can raise the leg on a stool for a leg, foot and ankle massage.

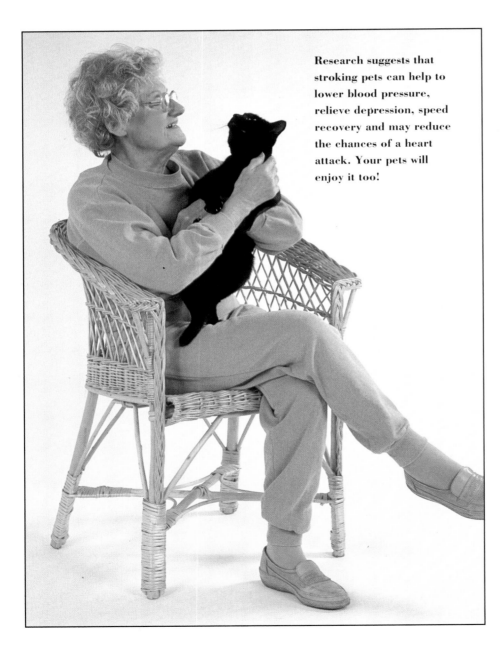

Research suggests that stroking pets can help to lower blood pressure, relieve depression, speed recovery and may reduce the chances of a heart attack. Your pets will enjoy it too!

Many older people suffer from aches and pains brought on by cold damp weather. A warm bath using aromatic essential oils such as lavender or sandalwood can comfort, soothe and relax you. Follow the bath with a gentle massage, and you will make headway in practising self-help. Massage stiff joints such as at wrists, knees, ankles and the hip. If the joint is affected by rheumatoid arthritis, massaging above and below the swollen area can relieve pain by relaxing the surrounding muscles. Avoid any swollen or inflamed areas.

The general wear and tear of joints which comes with aging is called osteoarthritis, and usually affects hips and knees in particular. Because the pain is often caused by the surrounding muscles, rather than the joint itself, massage can help to soothe the spasm and relieve pain. So long as the area is not swollen or inflamed you can massage the joint itself, working gently into the area which hurts most.

Massage can help to fulfil the deep-seated need for touch and communication, bringing psychological as well as physiological benefits, and contributing to a well-balanced lifestyle.

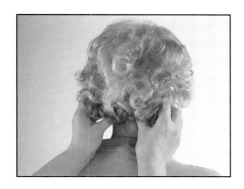

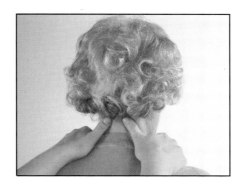

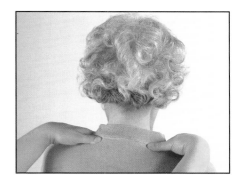

1 Start by gently resting your thumbs on the base of your partner's skull, just under the bony part. Relax your hands round each side of the head. Slowly and without too much pressure, slide your thumbs up through the hair, until you get halfway up the back of the head. Repeat three times, from the base of the skull to halfway up the head, to stimulate the nervous system.

2 Place the thumbs on the back of the neck and press gently, starting at the base of the skull and working down in a straight line toward the shoulders. This will loosen stiffness and relieve tension in the area. Repeat three times down the centre each time.

3 With your hand on either side of the neck, gently knead the tops of the shoulders, squeezing and releasing the muscles between your thumbs and fingers. Repeat three times the full length of the shoulder.

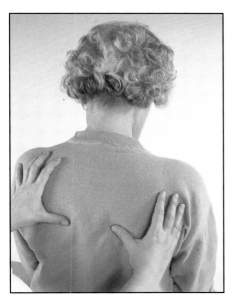

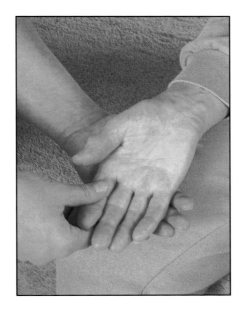

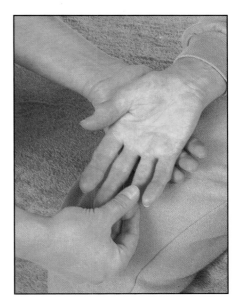

4 Bring your hands lower down the back near each shoulder blade, and use thumbs and fingers to massage upward over the shoulder blades, right up to the top of the shoulders. Slightly push into the back and release. Repeat from start to finish three times. You can vary the movement slightly by rotating the fingers as you work up.

5 Use any of the massage or self-massage techniques for the hands or feet, but avoid working directly on any joints inflamed with arthritis. Work above and below a swelling and then stroke up the limb toward the nearest lymph node. This stimulates the elimination of waste products and reduces inflammation.

6 If there are no signs of inflammation, you can use circular thumb movements all over the palm, then turn the hand over and work along each finger to the tip. Gently stretch each joint as far as it will go without causing pain, and then soothe the whole hand with firm strokes toward the wrist.

THE SENSUAL TOUCH

In the right circumstances, with a softly lit room, relaxing music, and using some of the more aphrodisiac essential oils such as rose, patchouli, neroli or sandalwood, a massage can be a highly pleasurable and sensual experience, relaxing the body and arousing the senses. Intuition will play a larger part in a sensual massage, as you discover which areas have the strongest impact on your partner's senses. It certainly isn't just the most obvious erogenous zones that bring pleasure – the back of the neck, scalp, solar plexus, inside of the elbows, hands and feet are just a few others.

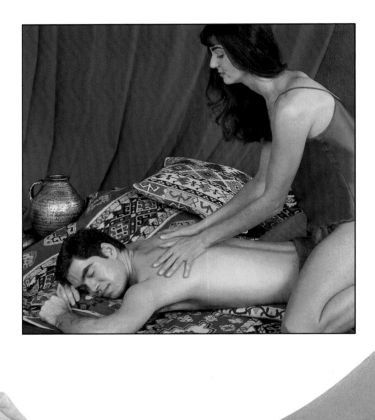

1 *With your partner lying on their front, start by resting your hands gently on the back of their shoulder blades. Fan the palms out across the back, sweeping your hands out and around over the shoulders.*

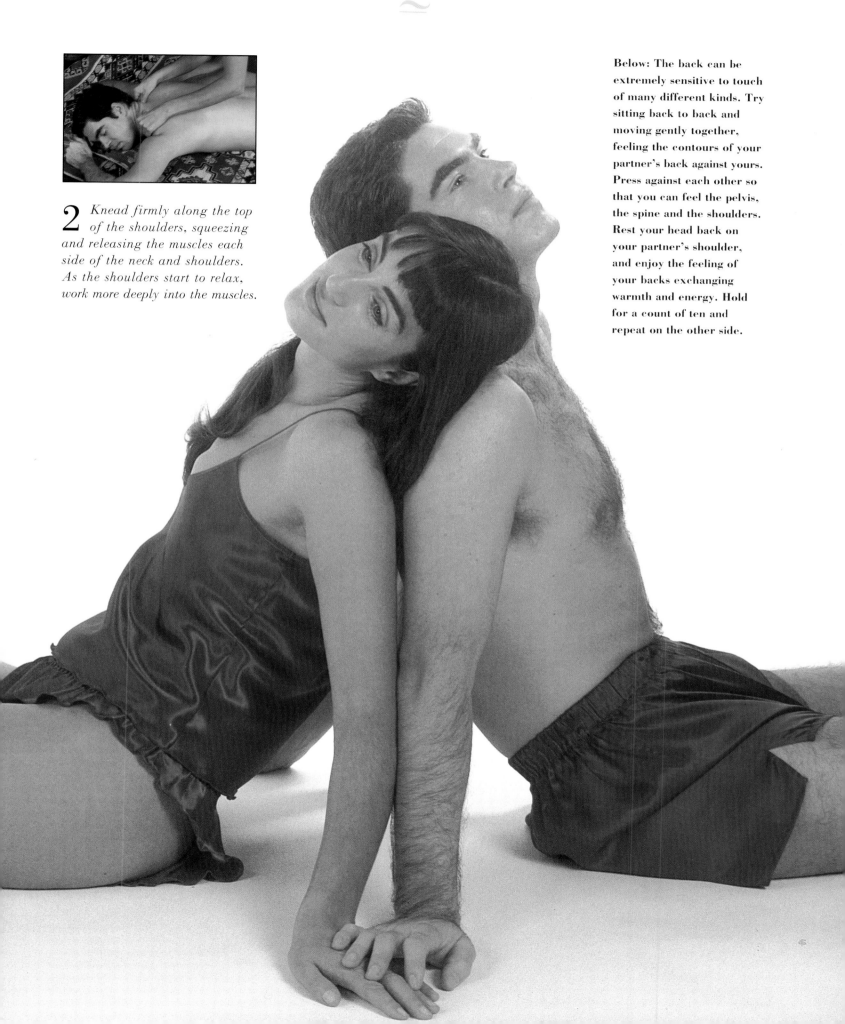

2 *Knead firmly along the top of the shoulders, squeezing and releasing the muscles each side of the neck and shoulders. As the shoulders start to relax, work more deeply into the muscles.*

Below: The back can be extremely sensitive to touch of many different kinds. Try sitting back to back and moving gently together, feeling the contours of your partner's back against yours. Press against each other so that you can feel the pelvis, the spine and the shoulders. Rest your head back on your partner's shoulder, and enjoy the feeling of your backs exchanging warmth and energy. Hold for a count of ten and repeat on the other side.

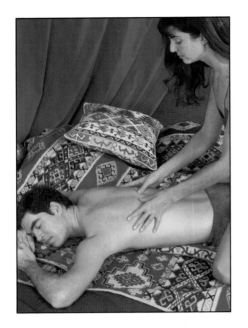 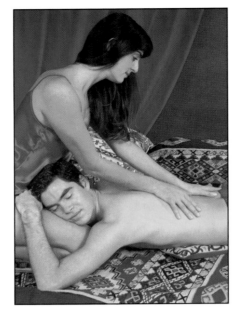 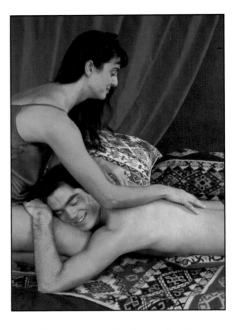

3 Check that your partner's head is still comfortable, then beginning at the nape of the neck let your thumbs gently stroke down each side of the spine. When you get to the lower back return up each side of the spine, this time working with slightly more pressure and rotating the thumbs to release muscular tension. Work up and down the spine two or three times.

4 Move round so your partner can rest their head on your thighs, and with long, effleurage strokes, massage the length of the back from the neck right down to the buttocks and back up the sides of the trunk. Repeat three times.

5 Starting at the lower back, gently stroke up either side of the spine, making light feathery strokes with your fingertips. Repeat three times, making the strokes lighter each time, until they can barely be felt.

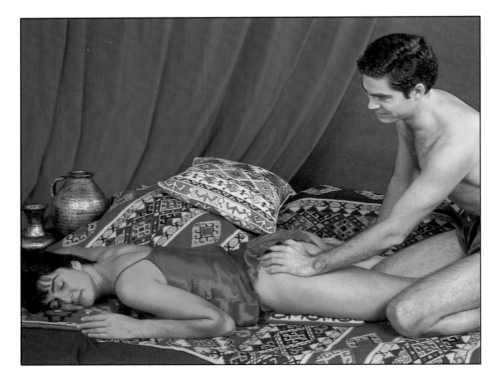

6 Left: Massage the lower back with some kneading. Using the flat, and in particular the heel, of the hand, knead the buttocks, then come back to the start and work over a different area. The nerves that cross this area relate to the man's groin, and the woman's uterus. The buttocks themselves are highly erogenous areas.

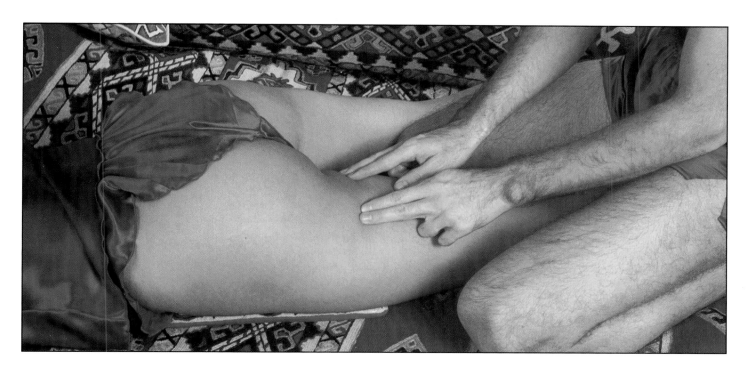

7 Curling your third and fourth fingers under, place your hands toward the top of the upper legs and circle your first and second fingers outward, one hand alternating with the other. This should be a slow, leisurely stroke with varying pressure.

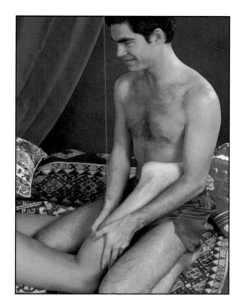

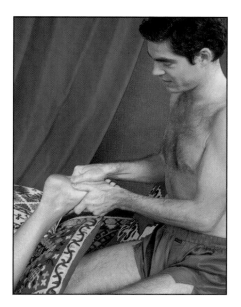

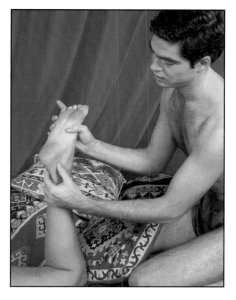

8 Support your partner's leg across your thigh and circle your thumbs over the calf, alternating the thumbs and applying firm pressure.

9 Raise your partner's foot, supporting its weight in your hands. Knead the instep firmly, using the thumbs to apply the pressure. Work all over the ball of the foot up toward the big toe.

10 Support your partner's foot in one hand, and place the thumb of that hand firmly over the centre of the instep. This has a wonderful, calming effect. With the thumb and first finger of the other hand, stroke round the ankle using circular movements.

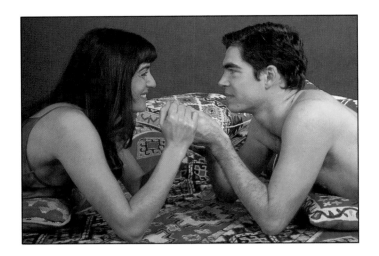

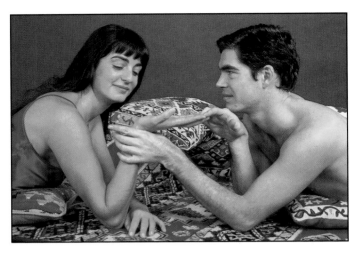

11 *At this stage, lie down facing each other, making sure you are both comfortable and well supported with plenty of cushions. Gently caress your partner's hands.*

12 *Gently stretch and release your partner's wrists, by flexing the hand backward and forwards. Softly stroke the inside of the palm with your fingers. Repeat on the other hand.*

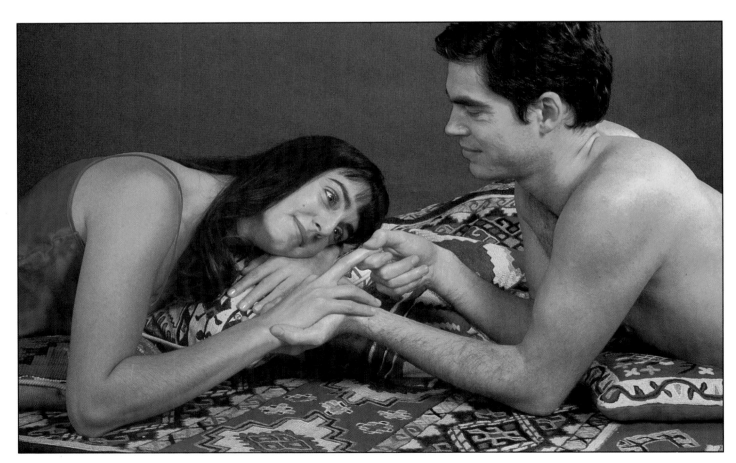

13 *Gently massage each finger, beginning with the thumb or little finger and working from the base joint to the tip. Try squeezing, rubbing and circular movements, and gentle pulling.*

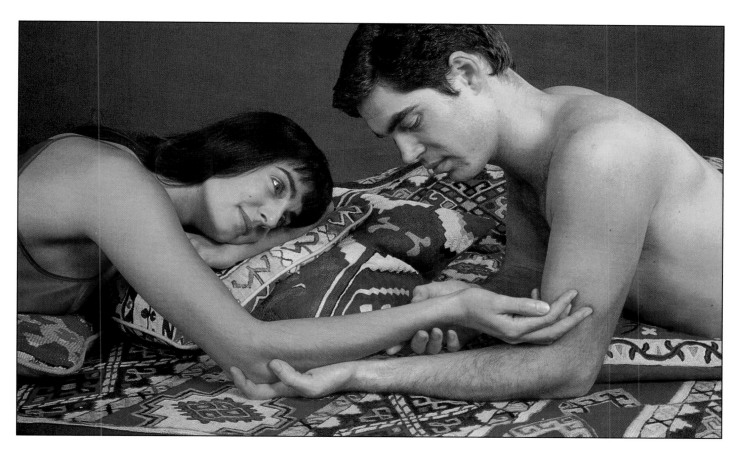

14 *Supporting your partner's elbow in one hand, use the other to caress and stroke the inside* *of the wrist just below the thumb, which is a particularly sensitive area. Continue working over the* *whole of the wrist area, using gentle circular thumb movements. Repeat on the other wrist.*

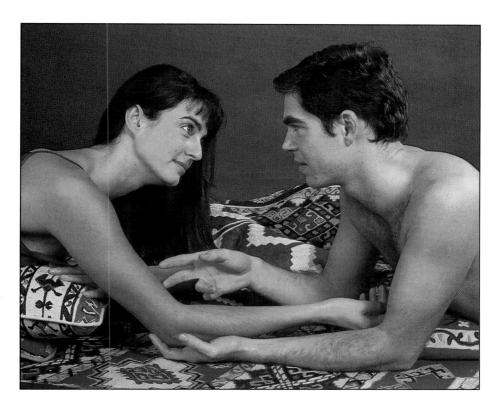

15 *Left: With feather strokes, use your fingers to stroke up the soft inner arm. This is a highly sensitive area when lightly touched and the effect is both stimulating and relaxing. Repeat on the other arm.*

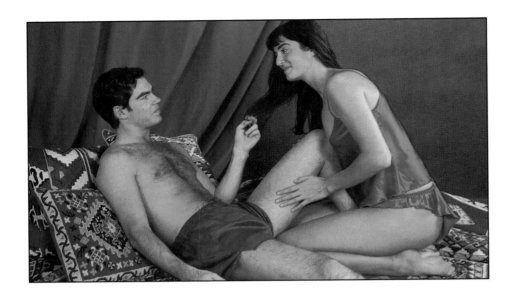

16 *Left: Use long effleurage strokes up and down the inner thigh area. Then massage closer to the highly erogenous region of the groin.*

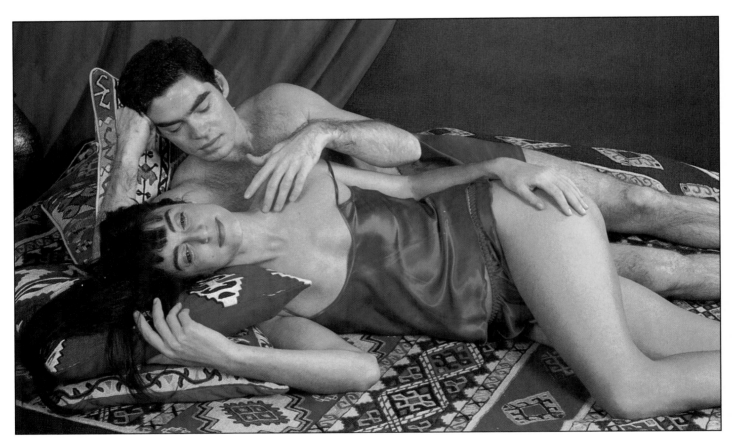

17 *With a feathery touch, stroke across the shoulders and up the neck, covering the sides, front and back. You can run your*

fingers up through the hair as well. Spend more time caressing the base of the neck, which arouses strong, sexual responses.

18 *Right: Finally, trace round the ear with your fingers, starting at the outside and circling toward the centre. Continue with soft pinching movements round the outside edge and on the lobe, where you will be triggering sexual responses from the adrenal gland and sexual organs.*

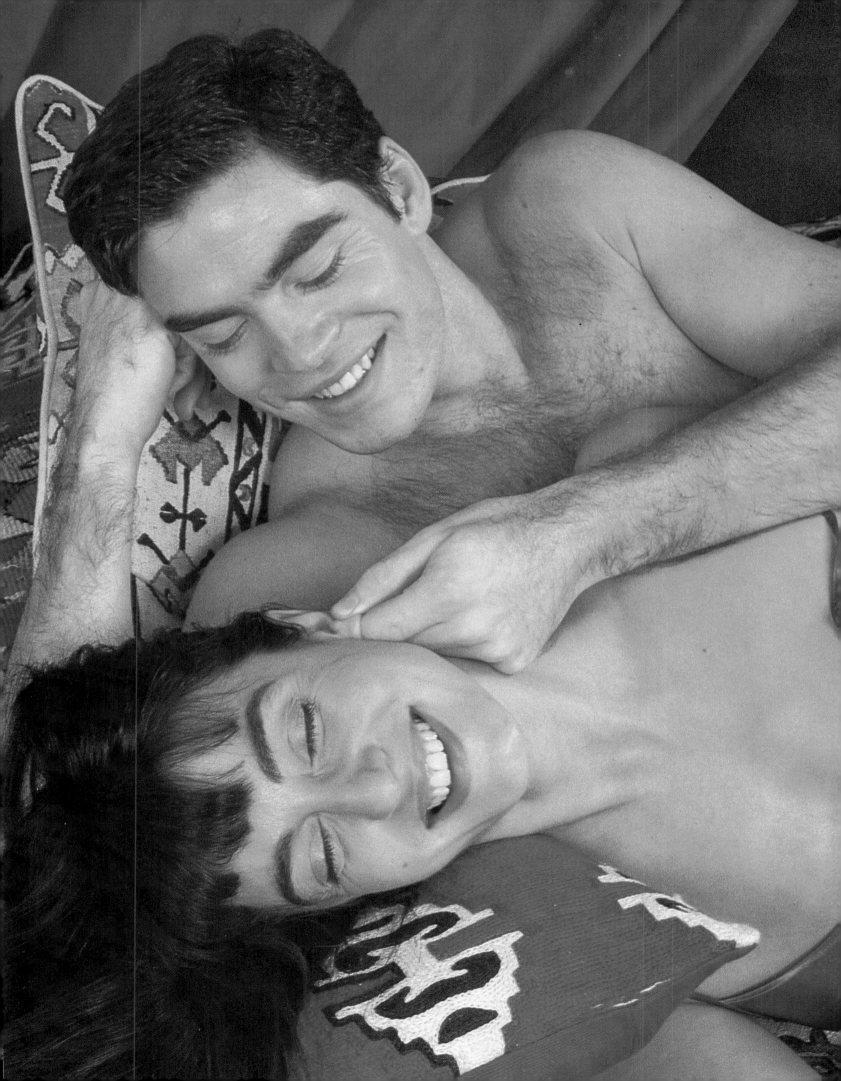

INSTANT MASSAGE

Sometimes, the idea of having tension in your shoulders and neck massaged away, without stopping to find the right place and the time to undress, is a particularly tempting one. There is increasing interest in learning how to do a shoulder massage with the minimum of disruption, especially in offices. Even at home, there are times when nothing is better than someone giving you a ten-minute shoulder and neck massage, in the comfort of an upright chair. There is no need to use oil if you prefer not to, and you can work through light clothing if simpler.

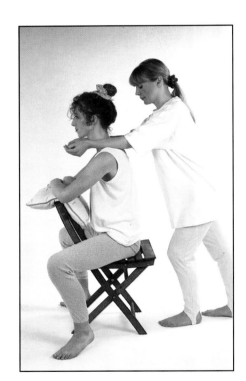

1 *Ask your partner to sit astride a chair facing the back. You can offer a folded towel or cushion for comfort. Standing behind your partner, begin by leaning on your forearms so that your weight presses down gently on to the fleshy part of the shoulders.*

2 *With your partner leaning forward, use* effleurage *strokes from the bottom of the shoulder blades, up the back and out over the top of the shoulders to finish at the top of the arms. Repeat four times.*

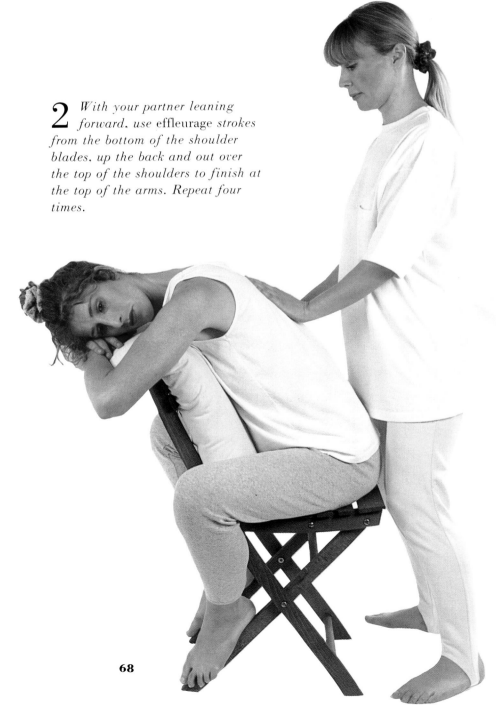

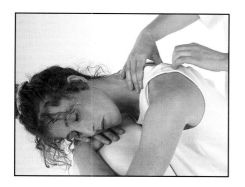

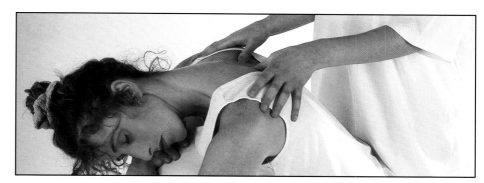

3 *With a firm* petrissage, *use both hands to knead out along the shoulders from the sides of the neck to the upper arms.*

4 *Starting as far down the lower back as you can, work up the spine with small circular frictions. Continue up the sides of the neck to* the base of the skull, then glide back down and work up again, this time moving out over the shoulders as you reach the top.

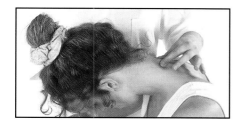

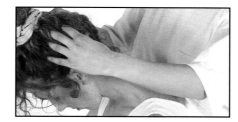

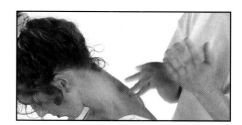

5 *Moving round to the side of the chair, tilt your partner's head forward and support it with one hand. With the thumb and finger of the bther hand, grasp the neck firmly and massage with circular movements, working up the neck and into the base of the skull.*

6 *Working from behind your partner again, massage the back of the head with both hands coming over the forehead and down to the temples with small circular pressures, moving the scalp against the skull. Lighten your touch at the temples.*

7 *First on one side and then the other, do some hacking across the fleshy parts of the shoulders and upper back, using the outer side of your hands to make short, brisk movements. Keep the wrists and hands very relaxed.*

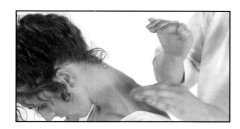

8 *Continue with a brisk cupping action across each shoulder, working on one side at a time.*

9 *Right: Finish the sequence by gently stroking down the entire back with one hand following the other. Repeat five times with each stroke getting lighter.*

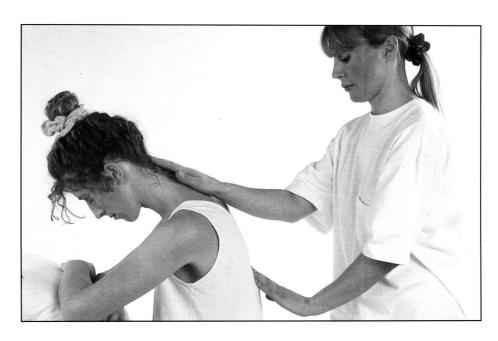

REFLEXOLOGY

ost people enjoy massage to the feet – one of the most sensitive parts of the body. All foot massage is beneficial and relaxing, but reflexology provides a more specific method of working to diagnose problems and stimulate health in the whole body. It is based on the principle that the body can be divided into ten vertical zones, each corresponding to an area of the foot, so that the feet are in effect a map of the body. A sensitive area of the foot indicates a problem in the corresponding organ of the body and by working on the appropriate trouble-spot, the larger problem can be helped. Reflexology can be an effective way of relieving pain and helping to restore the body's natural balance and well-being.

MAPPING THE BODY

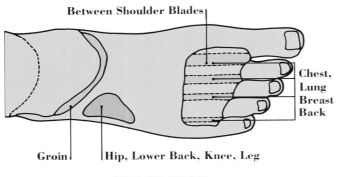

TOP OF FOOT

Between Shoulder Blades

Chest, Lung Breast Back

Groin

Hip, Lower Back, Knee, Leg

The feet provide an image of the body, with the head represented by the big toe, the inner arches as the spine, and the heel defining the pelvic area. The right foot corresponds to the right-hand side of the body and the left foot to the left, and the internal organs are then located in relation to the skeleton. Use the waist line and diaphragm as reference points.

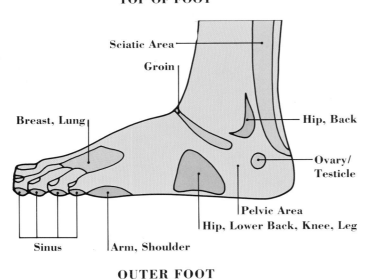

OUTER FOOT

Sciatic Area

Groin

Breast, Lung

Hip, Back

Ovary/ Testicle

Pelvic Area
Hip, Lower Back, Knee, Leg

Sinus

Arm, Shoulder

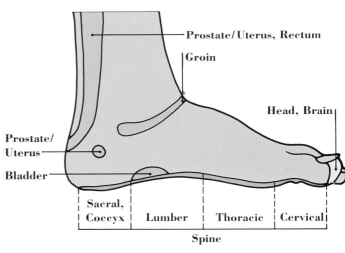

INNER FOOT

Prostate/Uterus, Rectum

Groin

Head, Brain

Prostate/ Uterus

Bladder

Sacral, Coccyx

Lumber

Thoracic

Cervical

Spine

THE BACKGROUND

The concept of using the body's reflexes for therapeutic purposes is not new – the early Chinese developed the technique of acupressure thousands of years ago. This provided the basis of knowledge about reflex zones and points and connections between different parts of the body. We know that the early Chinese, Japanese, Indians and Egyptians worked on the feet to promote good health, and many of the long-established principles developed by these civilizations are used in modern-day practice.

Reflexology as it is known today is based largely on the work of Dr William Fitzgerald and Eunice Ingham. Dr Fitzgerald devised his own system of acupressure points which produced an analgesic effect when stimulated. He found that the body could be divided into ten zones running from the top of the head to the tips of the toes, and that everything occuring in a specific zone of the body could affect the organs and other parts of the body in that zone. The theory was refined in the 1930s by a young physiotherapist called Eunice Ingham, who introduced a special grip technique and the action of the thumb on the foot and developed a more intricate zone system. Since then, the system has been further refined into the internationally recognized method that is practiced today.

Modern reflexology offers tremendous health benefits: it reduces stress, improves circulation, cleanses the body of impurities and toxins, and can revitalize energy levels.

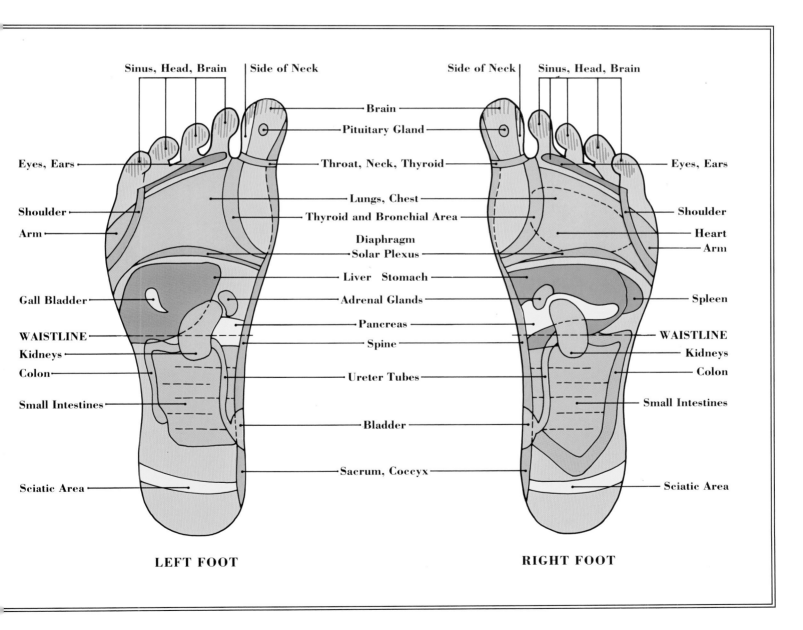

LEFT FOOT   **RIGHT FOOT**

BASIC REFLEXOLOGY TECHNIQUES

THE TREATMENT

Advanced diagnosis is a trained professional skill but some basic techniques can easily be used in a foot massage. You can also use them to work on your own feet, sitting with one ankle supported on the opposite thigh.

The following points will ensure a relaxing session:
● Work with your partner's foot in your lap or supported at the right height with cushions or bolsters.
● Your partner can sit in a comfortable chair with a footstool or small table to raise the feet.
● Ensure the back, neck and knees are properly supported, so your partner can relax completely.
● The massage is given without oil. You can dust the feet with talcum powder or work directly on the skin, if you prefer.
● Make sure your nails are short and well filed.

The following sequence of movements offers an introduction to reflexology. It is necessary to hold the foot correctly so that all points can be reached and stimulated with ease. The hands will swap their holding and working roles according to the part of the foot to be reached, so practice with both hands.

Apart from proper holding, the main principle to observe is leverage. Use the rest of the fingers in opposition to the working thumb to obtain more effective contact with the foot, or the thumb in opposition to the working finger in finger walking.

GREETING THE FEET

Below: The initial contact with the feet sets the tone for the whole treatment. Gently holding both feet relaxes them, allows you to learn about your partner and establishes a relationship.

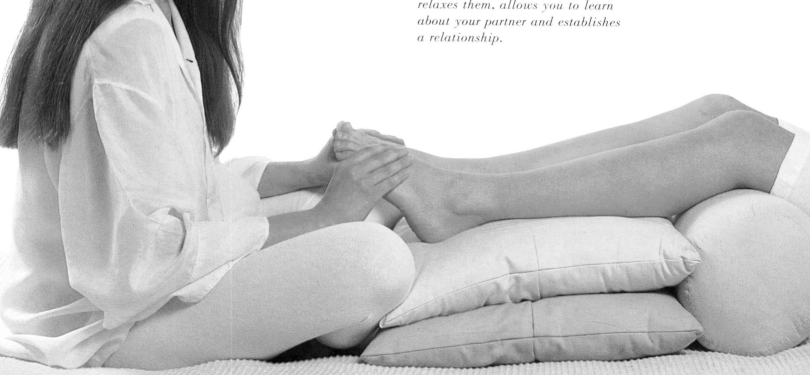

ANKLE ROTATION

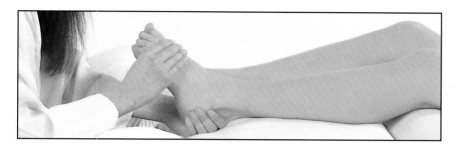

Begin with some relaxing movements. Stabilize the ankle by holding the right foot in the left hand, supporting the heel.

Gently wrap the fingers of the working hand below the base of the toes. Rotate the foot several times in each direction.

ANKLE STRETCH

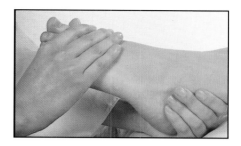

Using the same hold as for the ankle rotation, stretch the foot back and forth slowly to release tension in the Achilles tendon, taking care not to force the ankle joint. Then work all round the ankle, applying pressure. This area corresponds to the reproductive organs, legs and lower back.

SOLAR PLEXUS RELAXATION

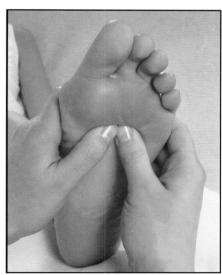

Place both thumbs on the solar plexus point located in the centre of the ball of the foot where there is a little indentation. This is a good relaxation exercise, particularly if your partner is very tense or nervous. You can also work on both feet simultaneously.

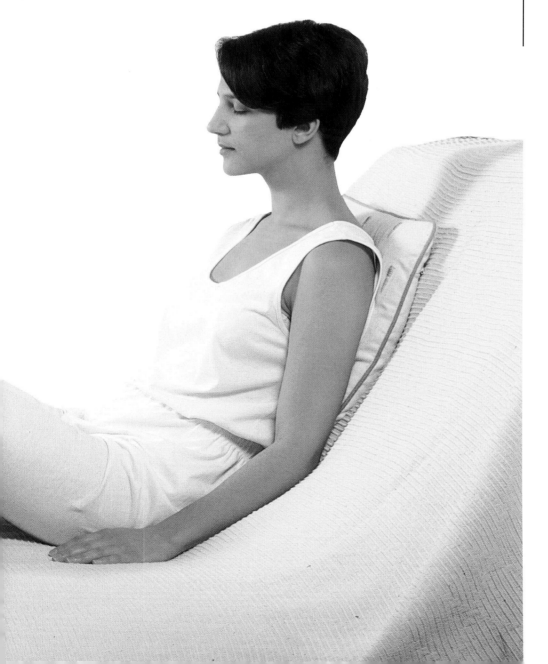

THUMB HOOKING

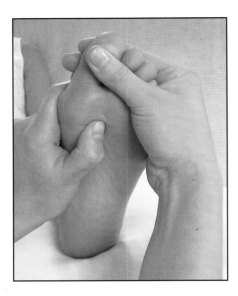

Place the outer corner of the thumb on a reflex point, with the thumb flat. Bend the thumb at the first joint to apply pressure, and pull back across the point. Use the other fingers for counter-pressure and raise the wrist to increase the pressure. Hooking is used to stimulate points that are too small for the walking technique (see right), such as the pituitary point, the solar plexus and lymph drainage points, and any point of soreness.

THUMB WALKING

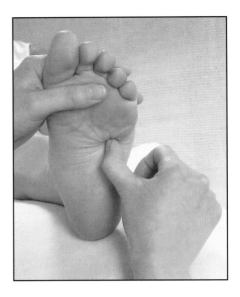

This is the principal technique for covering large areas. Thumb walking starts in the same way as the thumb hook and then the outside corner of the flexed thumb is rocked slightly forward. Maintain steady pressure as the thumb walks, avoiding an "on-off" movement. Press along the diaphragm line under the ball of the foot, then stimulate the spinal area along the main arch of foot from the heel to the big toe.

FINGER WALKING

1,2 *This technique is used to work on the top of the feet. The principle is the same as for thumb walking: flexing the first finger joint and rocking forward. With the holding hand, support and spread the toes, and push on the ball of the foot with the thumb of the working hand to provide leverage. Finger walk from the base of the little toe up to the ankle. Begin again, walking between the troughs of the next toes, toward the inside of the foot.*

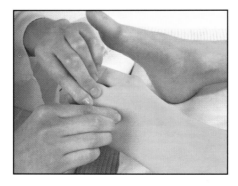
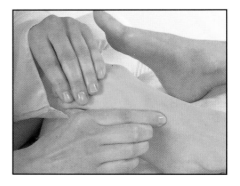

This helps to relieve tension in the chest and lung area, and the areas for lymph drainage and vocal chords which are located between the big toe and second toe at the top of the foot.

STROKING THE FEET

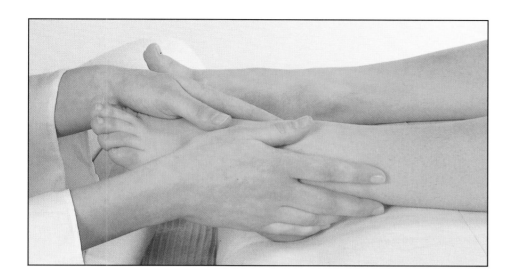

Left: Using alternate hands, stroke the foot softly from the ankles to the toes to smooth and relax the whole area of each foot.

DESSERT STROKE

Right: Take the foot in both hands and slide the hands gently up and down. Dessert strokes are enjoyable and can be used throughout the treatment to soothe and relax your partner after a sensitive reflex has been worked on. Always end the session with dessert strokes to rebalance the whole foot.

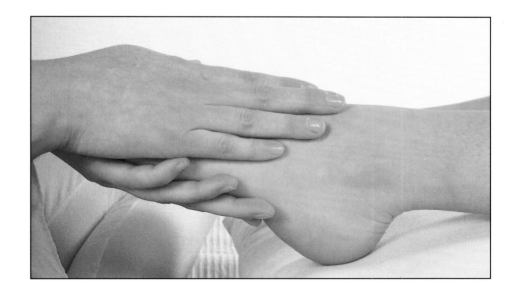

For an effective treatment:

● Explore the foot with the outside edge of the thumb, by the nail, but be careful not to dig with your nail.
● Make regular eye contact with your partner to check responses to specific pressures and to detect painful or sensitive areas.

● Pay extra attention to sensitive areas, which may feel granular, as these are usually due to calcification or deposits of lymph fluid. Work on them thoroughly to disperse the blockages and release energy in the zone.
● Work on each area of the foot several times and make sure that no area is left out.

● Work through each foot once to find sensitive areas and then a second time to reintegrate the foot and body.
● Join the movements and areas of the foot with dessert strokes.
● Always keep contact with at least one hand.
● Knuckling can be used to cover large areas of the foot.

THE AROMATHERAPY MASSAGE

An aromatherapy massage using essential oils is a therapeutic treatment for both mind and body which works mainly on the nervous system. Aromatherapy is both holistic and practical in that it helps to protect the body's life-saving immune system and energize or stabilize emotions. It is often called the "sensual science" because it combines the powers of touch with the sense of smell. More effectively than any other massage, aromatherapy can either relax or stimulate the body and mind. The highly potent essential oils penetrate the body via the skin and are also inhaled as the massage progresses.

SETTING UP

Any massage is relaxing but you can enhance the experience by following a few simple steps to help create the right mood.

An aromatherapist uses a massage bench, but at home you can work comfortably on a cushioned floor or a futon (Japanese mattress). An ordinary bed is not really firm enough. Prepare the floor or surface with a large cotton sheet covered with a bath towel. You should also have to hand a pillow, a large wrap-around towel for the body, and a warm blanket or even a hot-water bottle by the feet.

RELAXING YOUR PARTNER

Additional touches help to establish a calming atmosphere. You could fragrance the room with a burner, using a relaxing oil, and switch on some background music: play instrumental tracks, as voices can distract any train of thought.

The room temperature should be warm. Once the oils are gently massaged in, the whole body responds by slowing down and, although the skin may feel warm to touch, the body feels colder. It is important to keep your partner comfortable, so offer to cover parts that are not being worked on if you think your partner may be getting cold. Being at ease with one another is an important part of any treatment.

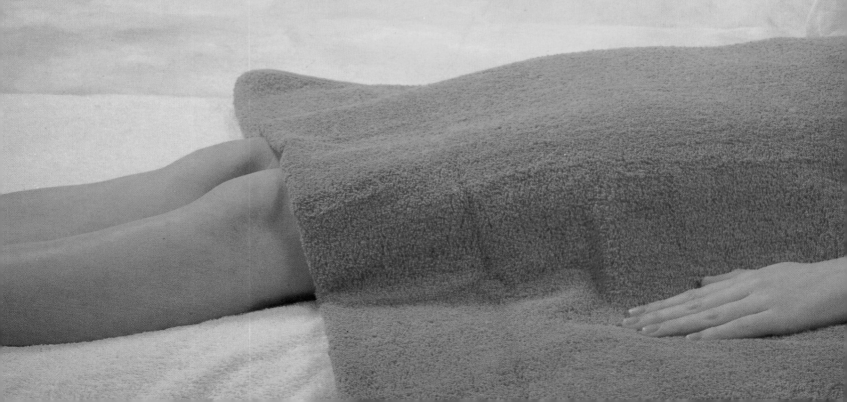

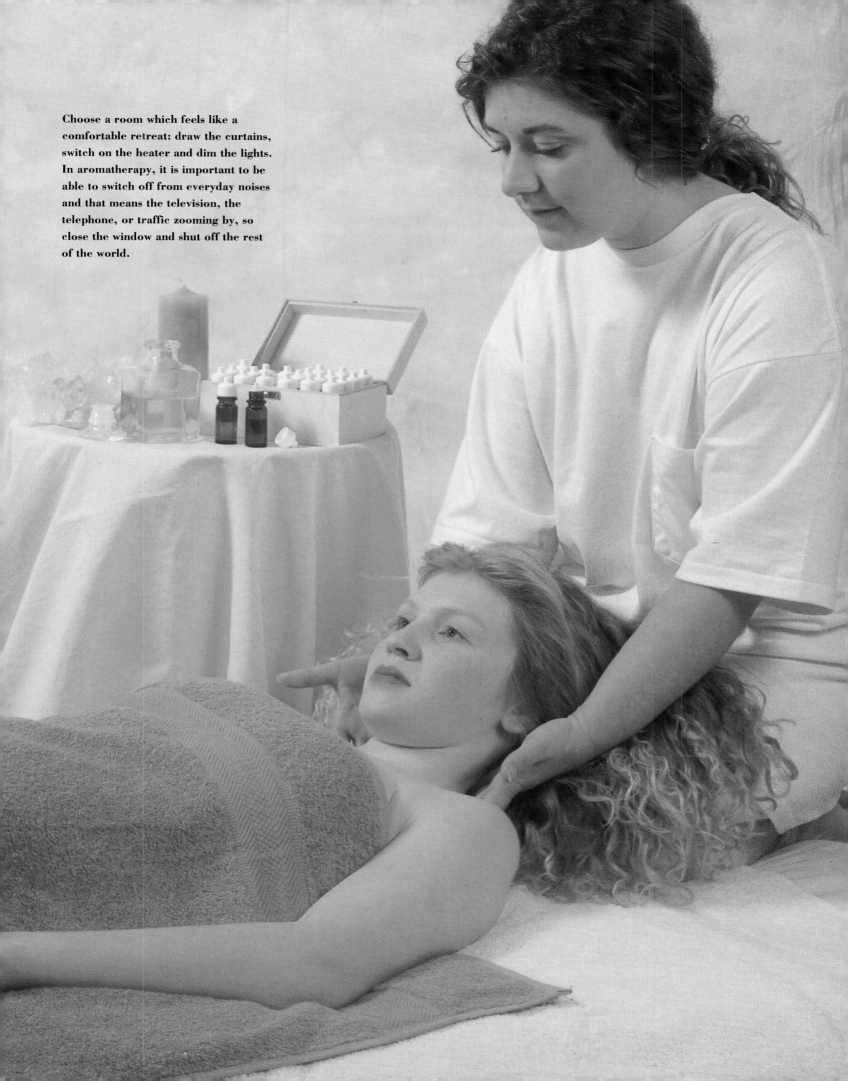

Choose a room which feels like a
comfortable retreat: draw the curtains,
switch on the heater and dim the lights.
In aromatherapy, it is important to be
able to switch off from everyday noises
and that means the television, the
telephone, or traffic zooming by, so
close the window and shut off the rest
of the world.

ABOUT THE TREATMENT

A complete aromatherapy massage takes just under an hour from top to toe. It is important to find out before massage about physical aches and pains, in particular back injuries, recent operations or whether the person you are massaging is in an "emotional" state of mind at the time.

GIVING THE MASSAGE

● Make sure you have read through the step-by-step instructions several times to familiarize yourself with the sequence. You don't want to keep stopping to refer to the book.
● Try out the movements on parts of your own body to get a sense of how the strokes should feel and how much pressure to use.
● Massage movements should be slow and gentle to help relaxation and eliminate tension which tightens the muscles.
● Remember that the movements should flow into each other. If you find you have missed out a step or gone on to the wrong part of the body, don't panic. Finish the part you are working on before going back to it, or leave it out altogether, rather than interrupting the flow of the massage.
● When you give the massage, make sure *you* are relaxed and comfortable, as well as the person you're working on, or you will transmit your own tensions to your partner and it will not be an effective massage.
● Try to maintain contact with your partner's body as much as possible; even as you move into a different position try to keep a hand on the body.
● When massaging different parts of the body keep the areas not being worked on covered with a large towel or blanket. The heat helps the body to absorb the oils.

CHOOSING THE ESSENTIAL OIL

romatherapists never start a massage immediately. In order to provide the most effective treatment, the therapist has to ascertain the state of mind and body of the individual, and establish whether there are any specific problems to attend to. Is the problem physical? Is it mental? Is it a combination of both? To help them to treat a wide variety of complaints, aromatherapists have many oils at their fingertips, but they never mix or use them until they have worked out a prescription for the receiver's individual needs.

Mixing the oils is a trained art, yet there are simple recipes you can use at home to deal with specific problems from muscular aches and pains to headaches and stress. With potent essential oils it is far better to use less, rather than more, so if in doubt, start the massage technique with a base oil like sweet almond and add two or three drops of just one essential oil. Lavender, rosemary and geranium are good all-purpose oils, or use chamomile for particularly sensitive skin.

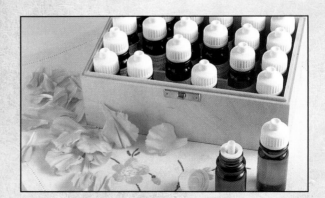

APPLYING THE OILS

 eep the oil in an easy dispenser or bowl so you don't have to worry about lids during the massage. But keep the oil covered in some way as essential oils will quickly evaporate.

● Always warm your hands before applying oils.

● Some therapists recommend warming the oil in your hands before applying it to the body as a courtesy to the recipient. Others advise against this on the grounds that it hastens evaporation of the essential oil and that the oil takes on your own energy rather than your partner's.

● If the part of the body you're working on is particularly hairy or the skin is very dry you will need to apply more oil.

● Keep your touch light and sensitive. Remember that your hands are the main channel of communication.

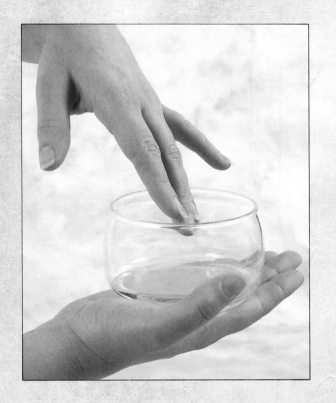

● If the recipient's back is stressed in any way, place a pillow under the knees when lying on the back, and under the pelvis when lying on the stomach.

● Wear loose comfortable clothing to give the massage, so your movements are not hampered.

● If oil is accidentally spilt on clothing, dab off quickly with a tissue. It will soon evaporate, but it may leave a stain so rinse out clothing in warm soapy water.

● For complete relaxation avoid chatting during the massage: play music if you don't like silence. But do encourage feedback from your partner – you must be told if something doesn't feel good.

● Ensure that the person you are going to work on is given the following set of guidelines.

RECEIVING THE MASSAGE

Before the Massage

● Have a cool shower or wash before a massage. Do not soak in a hot bath, or the oils will immediately seep into the skin.

● Don't use an underarm deodorant or body spray during the treatment, as this will block the effect of the oils.

● Don't have a large meal just before an aromatherapy massage as the body's systems will have to work too hard at digesting to be thoroughly relaxed.

● Don't drink alcohol before a treatment.

● Don't have a massage if you have flu or a fever or any serious condition (see Cautions). Wait until you are over the worst and

then let an aromatherapy treatment help restore your system's balance.

After the Massage

● Drink a glass of still water immediately after a treatment.

● Lie still for at least five minutes before getting up.

● Don't bathe or shower for at least twelve hours after a treatment to allow the oils to be absorbed by the skin and begin the all-important work of detoxifying the body.

● Drink plenty of water for the rest of the day as the kidneys will be active in eliminating the toxins.

● Avoid alcohol for at least 12 hours after the treatment to give the body a chance to detoxify thoroughly.

THE MASSAGE STEP-BY-STEP

Following your assessment, select the oils you are going to use and blend 10–15 drops of your chosen oils with four tablespoons of base oil.

The massage starts with your partner lying face down, with the back uncovered and the rest of the body covered with a towel or light blanket.

ESTABLISHING CONTACT

Take a few moments to create a bond of communication with your partner and to prepare yourself for the massage. Focus or "centre" yourself by becoming aware of your whole body and its role in giving the massage, and letting go of outside concerns to concentrate on the task in hand.

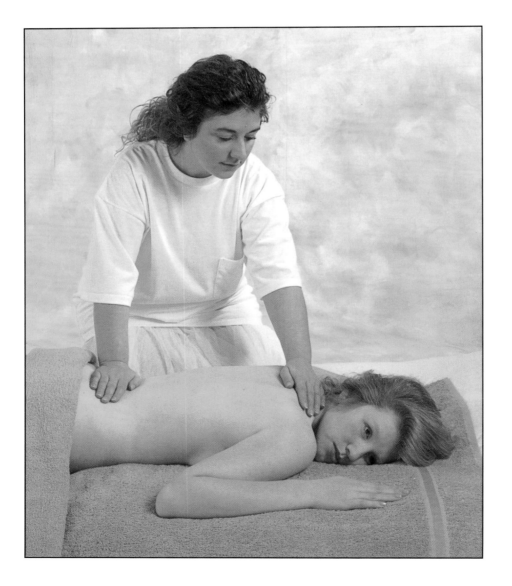

CAUTIONS

Aromatherapy is an holistic therapy in that it works on the person as a whole. Though it is an excellent way of treating minor ailments, stress and negative emotional states, it is not a substitute for conventional medical treatment. If symptoms persist, always consult a medical doctor.

Never attempt to treat the following conditions:

- cancer
- progressive neural disorders
- heart conditions
- advanced asthmatic conditions
- post-operative states
- severe varicose veins
- very high blood pressure
- epilepsy

For oils to avoid during pregnancy *see* Pregnancy Treatments.

Left: With your partner face down, rest one hand lightly at the base of the neck (the occipital bone) and place your other hand on the lower back (the sacral area). Hold the position for a count of 20, while you focus on your breathing and clear your mind. This is carried out with dry hands.

THE LEG

EFFLEURAGE (SMOOTHING STROKE)

This is a smooth, sliding movement which soothes the skin and distributes the oil. Always worked in the direction of the heart, effleurage improves circulation, lymph flow and the function of the muscles. It is used between movements throughout the massage to provide continuity and to prepare a new area with oil.

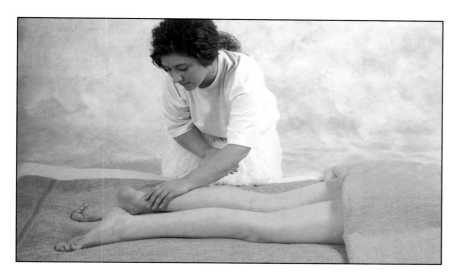

1 *Seated to the side of your partner, begin with one hand at the heel, brushing in an* upward, sweeping movement to the buttock ridge and sliding round to the thigh.

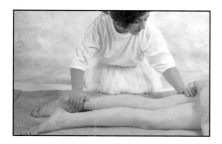 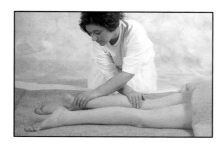

2 *As the first hand comes round the thigh, place the other hand at the heel and brush with an upward sweep, ending at the back of the knee.*

3 *As the second hand comes off, cross the first hand over and begin the movement again from the heel up to the thigh.*

Repeat the sequence about six or seven times, keeping the movements continuous and flowing, and then repeat on the other leg.

ANKLE THUMBING

The ankles are an important centre of energy, and this movement helps to relieve congestion.

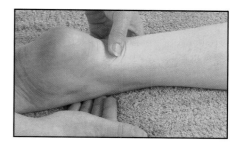

1 *Sitting at your partner's feet, cradle one ankle gently with your hands, allowing the thumbs to sit naturally above the heel.*

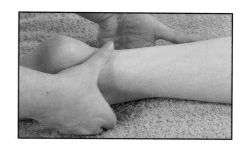

2 *Keeping the rest of the hand still, apply a light pressure with the thumb as it brushes in an upward and outward movement.*

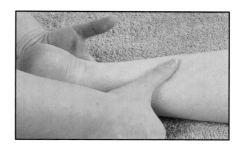

3 *Repeat with alternate thumbs, continuing in a rhythmic sequence for about 30 seconds.*

FLUSHING

*Flushing drains the lymph channels and stimulates the circulation.
This movement should not be used on anyone with severe varicose veins.*

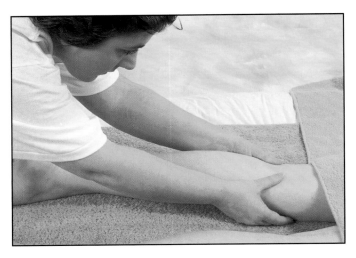

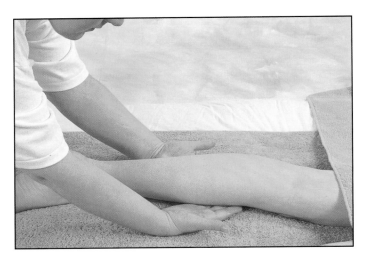

1 *Sitting at your partner's feet,
gently slide the thumbs up the
middle of the leg, ending at the back
of the knee.*

2 *Slowly bring the hands back
down to the ankles by brushing
down the sides of the calf muscle,
taking care not to drag.*

Repeat the movement five or six times.

KNEADING

*Move back round to the side of the leg for this movement. It is particularly
effective for relieving tension at the back of the legs.*

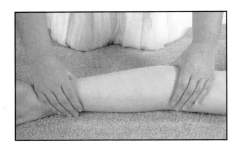

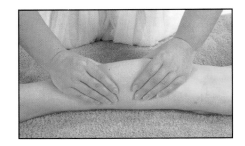

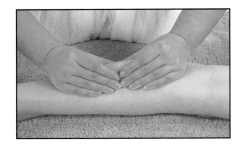

1 *Place the hands gently on the
calf, one at the top and one
just above the ankle.*

2 *Grasp the calf muscle firmly
with both hands and slide
them toward the centre of the calf,
lifting the muscle.*

3 *Using gentle pressure, knead
the area by bringing the
fingers and thumbs together and
raising the muscle further.*

Continue kneading for about 30 seconds.

WRINGING

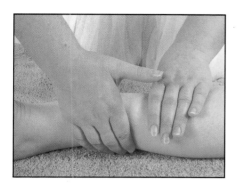

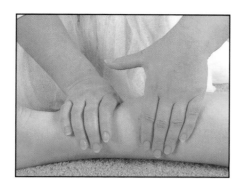

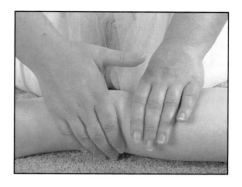

1 Place the hands on opposite sides of the calf, just above the ankle. Gently glide the hands past each other so the heel of one hand is pushing away from you while the other hand is pulling.

2 Keep the thumb of the pulling hand raised so the thumbs don't collide as they pass each other each time.

3 The hands alternate the pushing and pulling as you work all the way up the calf and down again. The pressure should be firm but gentle.

Clear these movements by flushing through again from ankle to back of knee.

THUMBING THE KNEE

This is the same action as the thumbing performed at the ankle base. It is helpful for people who suffer from cold feet as it stimulates the circulation.

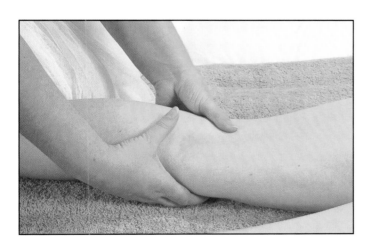

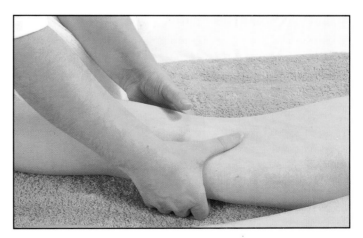

1 Cup the hands gently around the knee, allowing the thumbs to sit naturally on the fleshy part at the back of the knee.

2 With the same thumbing movement used on the ankles, brush one thumb upward and outward, covering the full width of the knee, and follow immediately with the opposite thumb.

FLUSHING

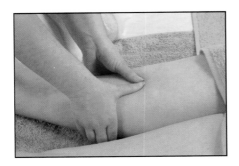

Flush through with the thumbs together from the back of the knee to the top of the thigh.

WRINGING

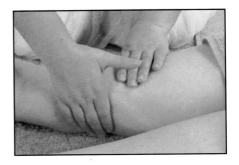

Wring the leg from the knee to the top of the thigh with the same action as used on the lower leg.

THIGH PUSH

This knuckling movement is very effective for breaking down cellulite, helping to disperse the fatty tissue and improve the circulation.

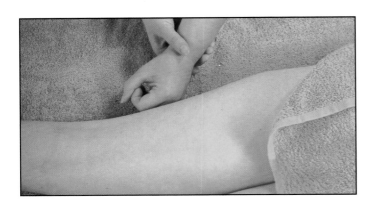

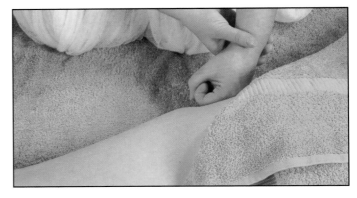

1 *With the supporting hand wrapped around the wrist of the working hand for stability, place the clenched fist on the side of the thigh, just above the knee.*

2 *Drag the fist slowly up the side of the thigh toward the hip bone. This is not a heavy action – all you need is gentle pressure.*

Repeat five or six times, working slightly different parts of the thigh each time.

Finish the leg massage by repeating the opening effluerage *movement and then repeat all the steps on the other leg.*

Cover the legs with towels before proceeding to the next stage. An extra blanket or hot water bottle at the feet might also be appreciated.

BACK MASSAGE

*The back carries a lot of strain and these relaxing movements are often
the most appreciated part of the massage. Don't be tempted to use too
much pressure: it is better to keep the strokes broad and flowing.*

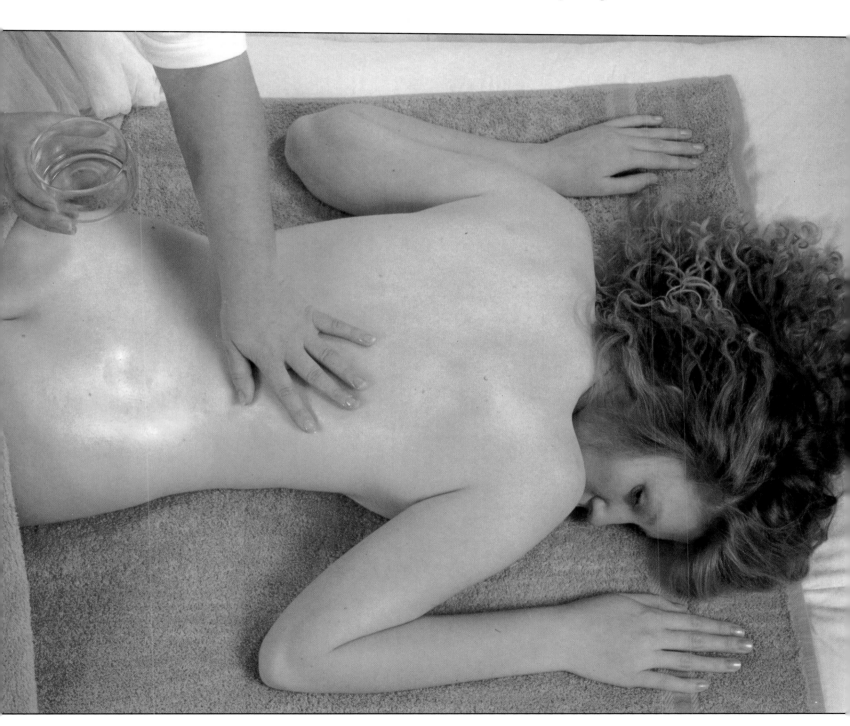

*Seated to the side of your partner, apply oil evenly over
the back with smooth upward strokes, following the
direction of the lymph flow.*

FIGURE-OF-EIGHT

This sequence loosens the tissue all over the back and helps to stimulate blood and lymph flow, and relieve tension.

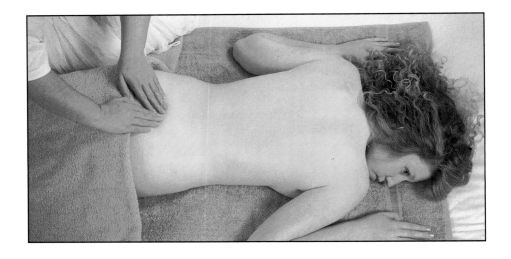

You should be kneeling level with the buttocks, facing the head so that you can lean into the movement and reach the shoulders without straining.

1 *To begin this large sweeping movement, place both hands on the lower back, just above the base of the spine, fingers pointing toward the head.*

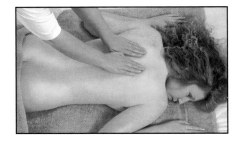

2 *Slide both hands all the way up the sides of the spine to just below the base of the neck.*

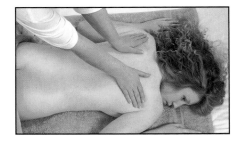

3 *Move the hands out around the shoulders and in toward each other across the upper back.*

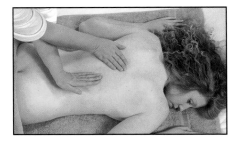

4 *As the hands pass each other, cross the right arm over the left and continue gliding.*

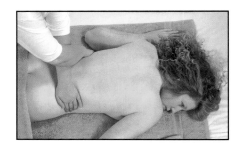

5 *With arms still crossed, reach down around the waist.*

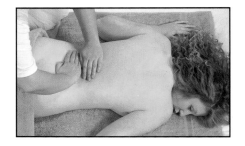

6 *Pull the flesh up firmly around the waist and then gradually release the sides as the palms glide to the middle of the lower back and pass each other.*

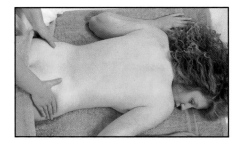

7 *Continue the movement by sliding the palms out around the hips and complete the figure-of-eight by returning the hands to the starting position.*

Repeat six times, always keeping the movements broad and flowing.

FANNING

This action works on the nerves along the spine and helps to disperse the fluid that accumulates in the back tissue as a result of tension. The effect is wonderfully relaxing.

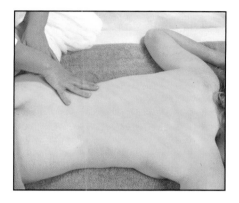

1 *Place one hand on the lower back, at the base of the spine. The fingers should be splayed open, with the index finger pointing to the side of the spine.*

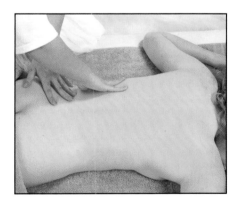

2 *Fan the hand round in an upward and outward motion away from the spine. The other hand follows on the same side as the first completes the movement. Work all the way up the side of the spine, alternating hands.*

Repeat the steps four or five times before moving round to work on the other side of the spine.

BUTTERFLY SHOULDERS

Before being given an aromatherapy massage, always wash off any anti-perspirant or deodorant. This is particularly important for this movement as it drains the lymph towards the major lymph glands in the armpits – the axillary glands. This movement relaxes the shoulder and disperses tension.

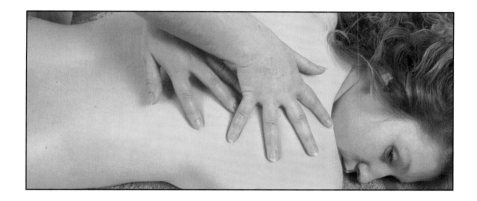

1 *Place one hand at the bottom of the shoulder blade (scapula) with fingers splayed and the second hand poised to follow on the same side.*

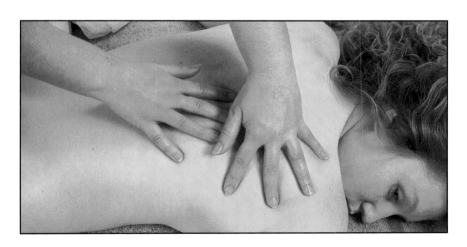

2 *Brush the hand up and out in a smooth fanning movement. Follow with the second hand, work all round the shoulder blade and out over the shoulder, toward the armpit.*

Repeat the whole movement four times, then work on the other shoulder.

FOREARM SWEEP

Kneeling at the side of your partner, turn the head away from you.

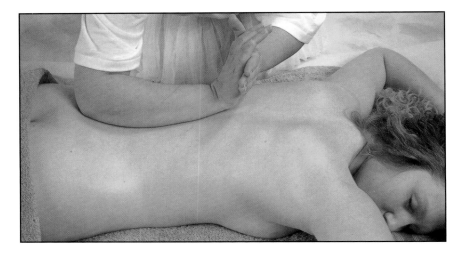

1 *Place your forearm alongside the spine with your elbow just above the buttocks. Clasp the working hand with your other hand for support and stability.*

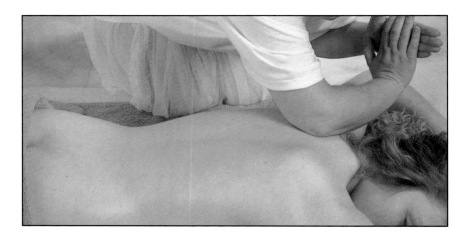

2 *Using the flat bone of the forearm (the ulna), slide all the way up the side of the spine to the top of the shoulder ridge.*

Lift the arm off gently and repeat twice from the beginning.

Then turn your partner's head and work on the other side of the spine, using the opposite forearm.

DRAINING

Sit to the side of your partner, facing across the back.

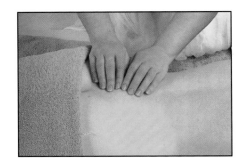

1 *With hands together and palms raised, place the fingertips at the side of the spine, just above the coccyx (tail bone).*

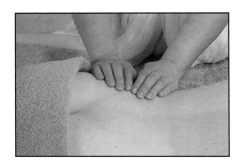

2 *Keeping the fingers together, pull them toward you down the side of the back.*

Repeat the movement all the way up the spine, ending at the base of the neck so the final movement pulls across the shoulders toward the glands in the armpit.

Repeat with the other side of the spine. You can work the opposite side without changing your position by reaching across and brushing away from the spine, or you can move around your partner and repeat as above, if it feels more comfortable.

KNEADING THE NECK

This gentle petrissage *movement releases tension and helps disperse the fatty deposits that can build up in this sensitive area.*

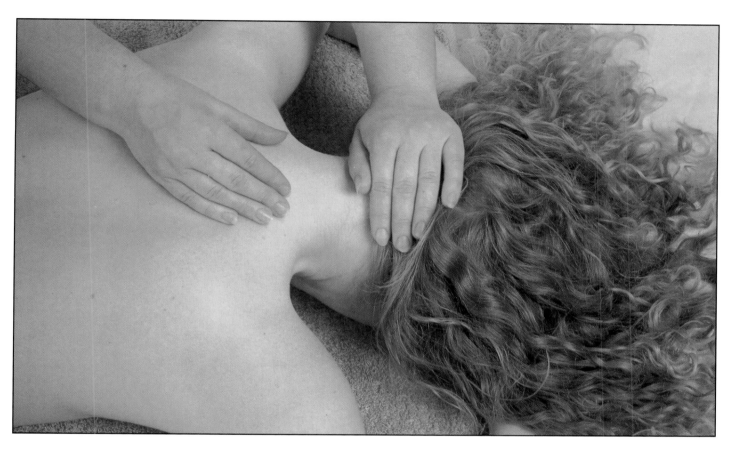

Your partner should rest facing down with forehead on hands, so that you can work your fingers into the base of the neck. Smooth the hair away from the neck.

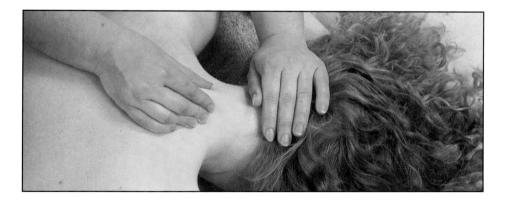

Resting one hand gently on the back of the head, use the other hand to pull up and knead the muscles in the base of the neck (the occipitals), rolling the muscle between the thumb and the other fingers.

FRONTAL MASSAGE

Help your partner to turn over onto their back, and ensure he or she is comfortable.
Provide cushions or rolled towels for any parts that need support,
such as behind the legs or neck. Cover the body up to the neck
with a towel or blanket to keep your partner warm.

SPINAL STRETCH

This movement is not suitable for people suffering from severe
back problems, though it helps relieve minor aches and stiffness.

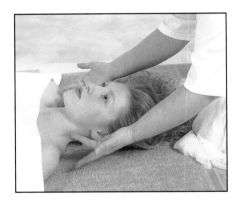

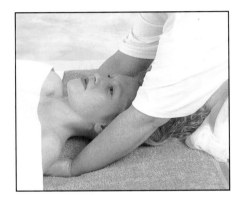

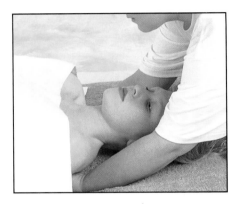

1 *Seated at your partner's head, place the hands to the sides of the neck, palms up, with the middle fingers lifted, to prepare for the movement.*

2 *Slide the hands underneath the back, just between the shoulder blades so the middle fingers are pressing on either side of the spine.*

3 *Gently lift the torso so the rib cage rises, maintaining the pressure from the middle fingers.*

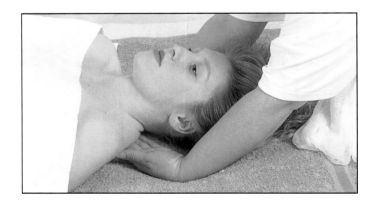

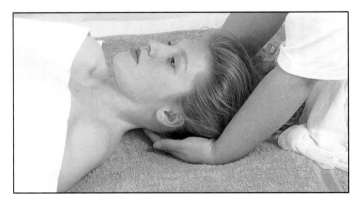

4 *Slowly pull your fingers up the sides of the spine. When you reach the top of the neck, hold for a count of two and then release. Repeat three times in all.*

5 *Finish the movement by cradling the head gently with both hands.*

THE FACE

This treatment is a great boost to the circulation, and the complexion will improve with each treatment.

Seated at the head, prepare the face for the massage with a simple refreshing cleanser, using upward and outward strokes. Apply a small amount of facial oil to the face and neck with flowing movements.

=====TAKE CARE=====

Even when diluted, essential oils are extremely potent so work carefully around the eye area. If the oil accidentally makes contact with the eye, apply a few drops of pure sweet almond oil to dissipate it. Never wash the eyes with water.

FOREHEAD STROKE

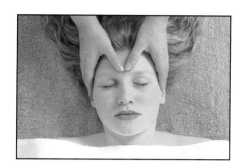

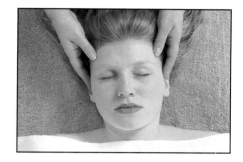

1 *Rest your thumbs on the centre of the forehead, just above the eyebrows, with the palms supporting the sides of the head. The stroke should be kept light and sensitive as the facial skin is very delicate.*

2 *Slowly draw the thumbs out toward the temples and down to the sides of the ears. Repeat the stroke several times, moving the starting position up a little each time until you reach the hairline.*

DRAINING THE CHEEKS

This sequence of raking movements stimulates the lymphatic flow in the face, improving the complexion, clearing the sinuses and releasing tension.

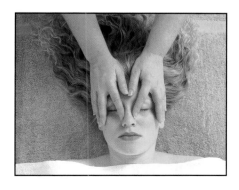

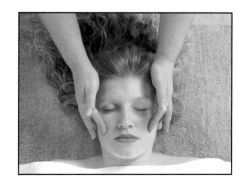

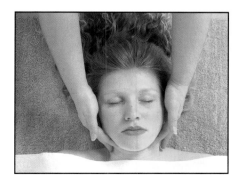

1 *Place the index fingers on either side of the nostrils and hold for a count of five.*

2 *Slide the fingers out and down to the ears. Lift the fingers and replace by the nostril. Sweep in a slightly narrower curve to reach the jawbone just below the ears.*

3 *Repeat with successively smaller curves, ending by tracing the laughter lines around the mouth, downward to the sides of the chin.*

CHIN MASSAGE

This not only tones the jawline, but also stimulates the energy points that govern the stomach and small intestine.

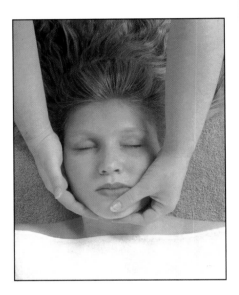

1 Place the thumbs on the chin, allowing the rest of the fingers to cradle the jaw.

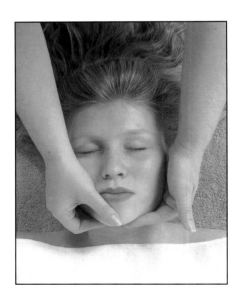

2 Brush alternate thumbs down and outward, with a light stroke. Repeat the movement six or seven times with each thumb.

NECK SWEEP

This is an extremely soothing stroke which improves the tone of the muscles as well as flushing the neck.

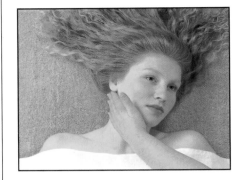

1,2 *Above and right:* Apply a little facial oil to the neck, upper chest and shoulder areas using the flat of the hand. Gently brush down with the hand from the side of the ear out to the shoulder, using a broad sweeping stroke to cover the area.

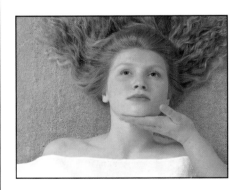

3 Repeat the movement working round the front of the neck, down from the chin to the top of the chest, and then sweep from the other ear to the shoulder.

The sequence of sweeps round the whole neck should be repeated three times.

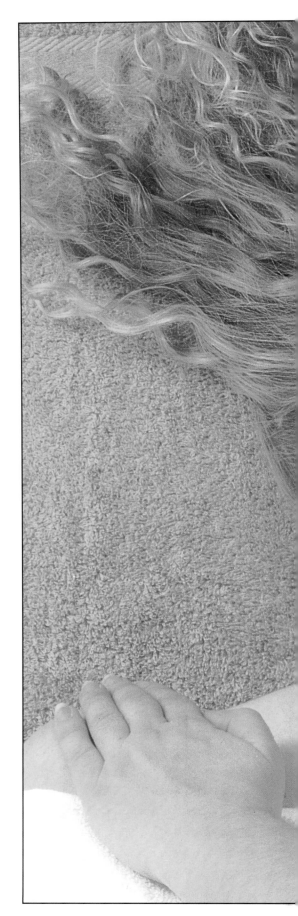

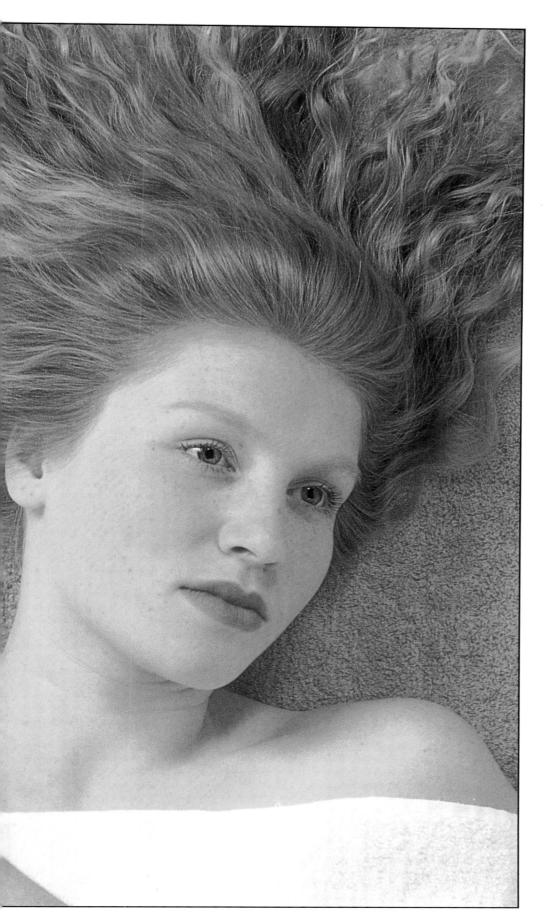

FANNING THE SHOULDERS

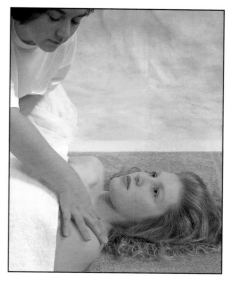

1 *With fingers spread, brush with the flat of the hand across from the breastbone and out over the shoulders.*

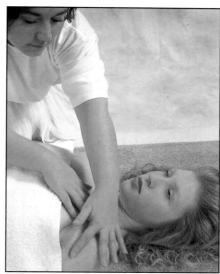

2 *The second hand follows closely behind the first, so they are draining simultaneously toward the armpit.*

Repeat twice before moving onto the other shoulder.

USEFUL ADDRESSES

MASSAGE

ORGANIZATIONS

Association of Physical and Natural Therapists
93 Parkhurst Road
Horley
Surrey RH6 8EX
Tel: 0293 775467

British Massage Therapy Council
9 Elm Road
Worthing
Sussex BN11 1PG

Institute for Complementary Medicine
Unit 4
Tavern Quay
London SE16
Tel: 071-237 5165

PRACTITIONERS AND COURSES

The Bluestone Clinic
34 Devonshire Place
London W1N 1PE
Tel: 071-935 7933

Champneys
Chesham Road
Wiggington
Tring
Herts HP23 6HY
Tel: 0442 863351

Henlow Grange
Henlow
Bedfordshire SG16 6BD
Tel: 0462 811111

Grayshott Hall
Headley Road
Grayshott
Nr Hindhead
Surrey GU26 6JJ
Tel: 0428 604331

London College of Massage
5 Newman Passage
London W1P 3PF
Tel: 071-323 3574

London School of Sports Massage
88 Cambridge Street
London SW1V 4QG
Tel: 071-233 5962

Massage Training Institute
24 Highbury Grove
London N5 2EA
Tel: 071-226 5313

Northern Institute of Massage
100 Waterloo Road
Blackpool FY4 1AW

American Massage Therapy Association
820 Davies Street
Evanston
IL 60201
USA

Boulder School of Massage Therapy
PO Box 4573
Boulder
CO 80306
USA

The Connecticut Center for Massage Therapy
75 Kitts Lane
Newington
CT 06111
USA

Australian Natural Therapists Association
PO Box 522
Sutherland
NSW 2232
Australia

South African Institute of Health and Beauty Therapists
PO Box 56318
Pinegowrie
22123
Johannesburg
South Africa

REFLEXOLOGY

The British School of Reflexology
92 Sheering Road
Old Harlow
Essex CN17 0JW
Tel: 0279 429060

British School of Reflex Zone Therapy
87 Oakington Avenue
Wembley Park
London HA9 8HY
Tel: 081-908 2201

International Institute of Reflexology
15 Hartfield Close
Tonbridge
Kent TN10 4JP

Reflexologists' Society
39 Presbury Road
Cheltenham
Glos GL52 2PT
Tel: 0242 512601

International Institute of Reflexology
PO Box 12642
5650 First Avenue North
St Petersburg
FLA 33733-2642
USA

FURTHER READING

MASSAGE

Nigel Dawes and Fiona Harrold, *Massage Cures*, Thorsons 1990

George Downing, *The Massage Book*, Wildwood House, 1973

Fiona Harrold, *The Massage Manual*, Headline, 1992

Tina Heinl, *Baby Massage*, Prentice Hall, 1983

Nitya Lacroix, *Massage for Total Relaxation*, Dorling Kindersley, 1991

Sensual Massage, Dorling Kindersley, 1989

Lucinda Lidell, *The Massage Book*, Ebury Press, 1984

Clare Maxwell-Hudson, *The Complete Book of Massage*, Dorling Kindersley, 1988

Sara Thomas, *Massage for Common Ailments*, Sidgwick & Jackson, 1989

Jacqueline Young, *Self Massage*, Thorsons, 1992

REFLEXOLOGY

Dwight C. Byers, *Better Health with Foot Reflexology*, Ingham Publishing Inc., 1983

Kevin and Barbara Kunz, *The Complete Guide to Foot Reflexology*, Prentice Hall, 1982

Laura Norman with Thomas Cowan, *The Reflexology Handbook*, Judy Piatkus, 1988

INDEX